"*Medicine at the Crossroads* is one of those many blessings given to us by Dr. Michael Attas, a physician, Episcopal priest, teacher, and more especially, healer. As a patient and dear friend for over fifty years, Dr. Attas has captured the very best of medicine in his time and has in such a discerning way defined its shortcomings. In a time of such radical change in the healthcare industry and when the very practice of medicine itself is drawn into question, Dr. Attas has shown us that the essential relationship is between the patient and the physician. For years Dr. Attas has been prescient about how medicine is changing and the role of physicians in that tide. At Dr. Attas' core is knowing and understanding the patient and his or her relationship to the physician in the midst of all this transition. The sense and deep understanding of Dr. Attas' humanity comes through time and time again in the stories of his patients. We can all benefit from his judgment and be greeted by his sense of balance when moving forward in this rapidly changing landscape. *Medicine at the Crossroads* reflects respect for science and technology and cautions us that science and technology must be greeted with the touch of caring and judgment about the human condition."

— UNITED STATES AMBASSADOR LYNDON L. OLSON, JR.

"*Medicine at a Crossroads* is a "stained glass" collection of short stories written for the primary purpose of starting a conversation about health care through the lens of the medical humanities in the delivery of care. Dr. Attas' forty years as a very successful cardiologist, teacher, and mentor—coupled with his being an ordained minister—provides him unique insights into the many challenges that modern health care faces today. His well-written stories are candid, transparent, and at times provocative as he describes his own journey in the field of medicine. His self-described and sincere approach to his life's work as a vocation rather than just an occupation or job allows him to share his personal feelings regarding the patient-physician relationship as a sacred bond that should not be unnecessarily broken by the advances in medical science and technology.

As an ordained minister, Dr. Attas is also able to provide a very thoughtful perspective relative to the spiritual role in healing as well as dealing with difficult issues such as death and dying. His insight into holistic medicine helps one to understand how the science of medicine and the art of medicine intersect. The last chapter of the book is an open letter to the reader that is a must-read for any individual considering entering the healthcare field as well as by those already serving.

Medicine at a Crossroads is insightful, challenging, and appropriately questioning what the future is for health care in America and how society must address some of the most important ethical questions surrounding the delivery of care now and in the future. I consider it a must-read. Thank you, Dr. Attas, for sharing these well-written, heartfelt stories."

— JOEL T. ALLISON, FACHE
Retired CEO, Baylor Scott and White Health
Senior Advisor, Robbins Institute for Health Policy and Leadership

"In the midst of the crisis of modern healthcare, Dr. Attas offers a new vision, reclaiming ancient wisdom, for what physicians are called to be. *Medicine at the Crossroads* is a deeply compassionate and humane book, overflowing with clinical and spiritual wisdom. It's not only a handbook about recognizing patients' needs in body and soul, but about how physicians, nurses, and anyone who holds the reality of life and death in their hands every day at work can start to recognize and meet his or her own needs of body and soul. This is a necessary read for anyone in health care committed not just to curing disease but to healing, both for patient and for the self. I hope every clinician will read it."

— KERRY EGAN, MDIV
Author, *On Living*

"*Medicine at the Crossroads* is about the intersection of faith and medicine, grounded in Dr. Mike Attas' forty years of practice as both physician and priest. Dr. Attas writes about the patient and practitioner, the physical and the spiritual, the sacred and the secular, the visible and the invisible—about joy and tragedy, about things both mundane and miraculous. Writing has been his way of grappling with the dilemmas and dissonances of modern medicine, with all its success and failures. His stories are both personal and prophetic. This is an important contribution to the conversation about the future of healthcare, reminding future healthcare professionals of their sacred duty to care for patients and urging us all to build a healthcare system based on compassion, wisdom, and justice."

— LAUREN BARRON, MD
Director, Medical Humanities Program, Baylor University

"In carefully crafted vignettes, Doctor Attas reveals the beating heart of medical practice: the life and death stories patients willingly share and to which the physician must respond. He knows—and shows—from much experience the crucial differ-ence between curing and healing, and how the latter remains possible even when the former is not. The reader will find hard-won wisdom on every page."

— BRIAN VOLCK, MD
Pediatrician and Author,
Attending Others: A Doctor's Education in Bodies and Words

"Dr. Mike Attas, cardiologist, Episcopal priest, and professor of Medical Humanities, has spent much of his professional life thinking about the differences between curing and healing, the complexity of moral decision-making, and the role that intel-ligent faith can play in those decisions. He has been a teacher for his patients and families of patients, for parishioners, for pre-med students, and for those of us who have engaged him in conversations about medical decision-making. *Medicine at a Crossroads* extends to a wider audience the opportunity to encounter Attas' compassionate wisdom. He is particularly insightful concerning the ever-changing technological and economic environment within which medicine is practiced in the twentieth-first century."

— ROBERT BAIRD, PHD
Emeritus Professor of Philosophy, Baylor University

"Touching, real-life experiences and a relevant point of view on health care."

— JIM TURNER
Former Chairman, Baylor Scott and White Health System

"This is a heart-felt, hopeful collection of essays from a physician who knows a lot about hearts and hope. The deep humanity, faith, and compassion represented in them echo the singular contributions he has made to the education of so many aspiring doctors. Attas generously allows us all to savor not only the formative privilege of being present for the wrenching, wonderful realities of human suffering and death, but also the profound and humane wisdom to be gleaned there, wisdom that informs each word in this remarkable book."

— MARGARET MOHRMANN, MD, PHD
Professor Emerita of Pediatrics, Medical Education, and Religious Studies at University of Virginia and Author, *Medicine as Ministry*

MEDICINE at the CROSSROADS

A Collection of Stories and Conversations to Forge a Vision for Health Care

Michael Attas

Michael Attas, MDiv, MD

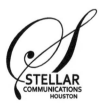

STELLAR
COMMUNICATIONS
HOUSTON

Medicine at the Crossroads
A Collection of Stories and Conversations
to Forge a Vision for Health Care

Published in the United States of America

Paperback ISBN 978-1-944952-22-8
E-book ISBN 978-1-944952-23-5
Library of Congress Control Number 2018956787

Stellar Communications Houston
www.stellarwriter.com
281-804-7089

To my wife, Gail.

This project could not have been born nor come to fruition without your love, support, and feedback. When my stamina and emotional energy would fade, as it does in medicine, you were always there to guide me and gently nudge me back on track. We all have our own dark nights of the soul. You helped me through mine. This book is dedicated to you, your wisdom, and your spirit.

"Telling a story is like reaching into a granary full of wheat and drawing out a handful. There is always more to tell than can be told."

— WENDELL BERRY, *JAYBER CROW*

CONTENTS

FOREWORD BY JUDGE KEN STARR

In the spring of 2010, I found myself in a condition highly characteristic of contemporary life—transition. In typical American fashion, I was pulling up stakes in one region (California) and being drawn elsewhere as a magnificent opportunity beckoned — to serve as the fourteenth president of Baylor University in my native Texas. The transition process that rapidly unfolded was at once inspiring and daunting. With its storied history boasting a founding during the long-past days of the Republic of Texas, Baylor was by my lights an admirably vast institution with a presence—through its programs and people—literally around the globe. It was humbling to listen and learn.

High on the "must do" list put before me was to meet Mike Attas. As the new boy on the block, I was instructed that I needed to learn about one of the University's academic jewels, a relatively new program that embodied the noble spirit of an unapologetically Christian university. I was to meet the founder of Baylor's program in Medical Humanities.

This rookie president soon found himself ushered into the presence of Michael Attas, M.D., a renowned cardiologist, teacher, mentor, Episcopal priest, fly fisherman . . . on and on the staggeringly-impressive list of interests and accomplishments continued. Sitting in my new office at Pat Neff Hall on Baylor's gorgeous campus situated on the banks of the Brazos, I learned immediately that this modern-day polymath was not only charmingly winsome, but he was also deeply empathetic. He connected with his somewhat daunted host in a deep, powerful way, a physician-priest of obvious humanity. "He must have a world-class bedside manner," I thought. As if more were needed, it turned out that in his own student journey at Baylor, Dr. Attas had not only performed brilliantly in the classroom and laboratory, he had played football in the days of the old Southwest Conference. A man for all seasons, not only autumn on the gridiron, Mike Attas immediately entered my pantheon of Baylor giants, past and present.

True, the University had produced governors, virtually countless legislators and judges, both federal and state, and thousands of pastors, physicians, teachers, missionaries and business leaders. But as I learned more about the ideas informing the founding of Medical Humanities and its brilliant implementation, I identified Mike Attas as one of the University's most transformational and inspiring alumni.

Dr. Attas's uplifting, deeply moving book captures and conveys powerfully the ethos of what makes the Baylor family "Baylor Proud." Mike has collected stories from his own vast reservoir of experience that will both educate and inspire. These tales of truth will draw a smile, and occasionally a tear, as the stories cascade toward a compelling conclusion—medical science and technology must be accompanied by a deeply caring and compassionate humanity, richly informed by art, literature, philosophy, and religion. Laughter heals; so do therapy dogs, but so does prayer—which heals even when it does not cure.

The structure of Dr. Attas's narrative demonstrates the extensive body of wisdom gained through his life of highly successful clinical practice, enriched deeply by his extensive reading and prayerful reflection—as well as his formal theological training. The book's organizational emphasis is on "The Physician," while attending dutifully to "The Patient" and, as its capstone, "The Healthcare System."

As Dr. Attas's poignant stories unfold, the reader will continually be transported back to memories of his or her own life experiences, or perhaps in the case of undergrad and medical students just beginning their adult-life journeys, to recollections of stories gleaned from sitting around the family table, or listening to the voices of grandparents or favorite aunts. Each story Dr. Attas recounts in this illuminating compendium is a modern-day parable, pointing the way to an enduring truth about the human condition.

Especially moving are his riveting stories of end-of-life dramas, such as the rancher whose will to live gave him, by God's grace, one last bluebonnet-filled spring, with new-born calves and flowering pasturelands symbolizing the chapters of well-lived lives, supported by loving families gathered around to bid farewell on this side of eternity. On a happier note, the story of the miraculous recovery of the patient deemed dead only to experience, Lazarus-like, a complete recovery, the takeaway is this: humane instincts guided the wise physician to follow his life-affirming judgment, rather than accept the grim reality suggested by the most sophisticated medical devices available in our advanced economy. Yet, as his analytical mind surveys the horizon of our broken healthcare system, Dr. Attas searingly critiques the wasteful folly of budget-busting extravagances—wasteful expenditures at the end of life's journey, while casting aside the immeasurable value of counsel and support—the overarching value of presence.

How fitting and proper, as Mr. Lincoln would say, that Dr. Attas's book of wisdom and discernment opens with a note of admiring thanks from one of his former students at Baylor. Allison—now a successful and wisdom-filled clinician—writes this: "The philosophy, literature, and ethics courses founded by Dr. Attas at Baylor University were by far the most important of my education—more than any of the sciences in the premed coursework." So too, during my six years of service at our beloved Baylor University, no program proved to be more inspiring and affirming of what higher education should be than Medical Humanities—the proverbial house founded on solid rock, the house that, by God's good grace, my treasured friend Mike Attas built.

A PERSPECTIVE FROM A PHYSICIAN-IN-TRAINING

As an early medical student, I felt that my Medical Humanities major needed an explanation, sometimes even an apology.

"Oh, but I minored in Biology and Chemistry," I would say.

I realize now that this perceived "weakness" is, in fact, a tremendous asset. Majoring in Medical Humanities was the absolute best decision for me. The philosophy, literature, and ethics courses founded by Dr. Attas at Baylor University were by far the most important of my education—more than any of the sciences in the pre-med coursework.

It was in these classes with Dr. Attas that I first learned about medicine through stories. I learned about how patients experience illness and suffering, how physicians cope with stress and loss, and how these two protagonists come together to find healing in the absence of a cure as well as harmony in the presence of chaos. I learned about the physician-patient relationship and the physician's role in helping patients negotiate the more difficult pages and chapters of their lives.

My patient care experiences in clinical rotations proved that there is something to learning about stories first and science second. Even the order in which we conduct a History and Physical Exam bears this out. Seeing a patient as a person within a narrative before a diagnosis and a problem list sets the stage for enhanced understanding, improved care, greater trust, and better outcomes.

Today, I am helping to write some of my patients' stories and even revise a few endings. I have encouraged one patient not to let her uterine prolapse restrict her ability to work and to opt for a much-needed surgery. I have held another patient's hand while she tearfully stared at an ultrasound screen and wrestled with the decision to accept intervention for her twins. As an obstetrician/gynecologist, I've always known that it is a gift to be a part of a woman's personal narrative, but these patients have shown me how to best receive it.

I am who I am because of the lessons of Dr. Attas. He is a physician, teacher, and mentor who passionately loves and follows the Lord, a shining and needed example for this young pre-med student. He empowered me to boldly live out my faith in an academic environment where, for the first time in my life, I found myself in the minority as a Christian. I continue to carry this with me on this journey that truly is a calling and a privilege. Thank you for everything, Dr. Attas.

Allison Sellner, MD
Obstetrics & Gynecology
Baylor College of Medicine, Class of 2018
Graduated with Highest Honors

INTRODUCTION

For centuries, stained glass has captured the human imagination through its power to convey beauty and the incredible depth of the human story. One impossibly small fragment at a time, each piece of light and color has been hammered and layered together to create a glass pane. Each pane, in turn, has been forged into a scene of biblical times or human history. And when light has poured through the stained glass scenes, a larger narrative truth has emerged that extends beyond the bounds of time and space.

For me, medicine has the same ineffable power. It draws me out of myself and into the wonder of another story.

At the heart of medicine lies a singular and very powerful human story. It can be the story of brokenness, grace, redemption, and healing. It can be the story of unbearable pain and unrealistic expectations. It can be the story of beauty that inspires, moves, and creates a new being. It can also be the story of failures—the story of mistakes, pain, suffering, loss, and death. It is all of the above, for it is our story. For better or worse, it is the story of all of humanity.

And so it is with medicine today. Ours is a time in which medicine is being scrutinized, debated, transformed, and criticized—and rightly so. Some of us sense that we are on a national train headed toward a disaster of healthcare delivery. Too many are left out, costs are escalating, and it seems that the system is unraveling before our very eyes. Meanwhile, polemic anger is dividing all of us.

This I know: we are standing at a crossroads. The old system is breaking down, but we don't have a good new one to replace it. And in my own moments of anguish, despair, and cynicism as a physician, I have joined the throngs who cast stones at my calling.

But I also know that I have never wished to do something different with my life. Medicine has brought me to my knees in gratitude and reduced me to tears more than I care to remember. It has humbled me, broken me, hurt me, lifted me, and healed me. It has left me both confused and enlightened, wounded yet standing, sad yet hopeful.

It is with this hope that I submit that we need to return to an older way—a way as ancient and sacred as a stained glass window. We need to return to the individual panes of glass in the larger work of art, for medicine is and always will be an art form.

I realize this goes against the grain. As pundits call for a new way of practicing medicine, I agree that change is an inevitable part of the human journey and that technology should be embraced and utilized. But technology and science will not sustain us in the times ahead in medicine.

And it seems that some people agree. Much to my surprise, in 1999, Baylor University welcomed the idea of an "experimental" program in Medical Humanities. It would redefine how students prepared for a career in health care by providing classes on Spirituality and Health Care, Philosophy of Medicine, Literature and Medicine, Economics of Health Care, the Nature of the Patient/Physician Relationship, and a few other equally esoteric courses and subjects. I had just completed a masters of divinity degree when I founded the Medical Humanities Program, and I didn't know that I was about to start a journey that would change the trajectory of my life.

As I began to teach, I found that the stories collected in the basement of my mind bubbled to the surface. Many were raw and recent, while others were so old that names and places were forgotten. But all of the stories had entranced and shaped me, and their essence was embedded in my soul. They were stories that had resonated with me when the staleness of electronic medical records had left me empty, and now the Greek storyteller in me had finally found a voice for them.

To my even greater delight and surprise, the students accepted my challenge to think about medicine in a different, non-scientific way. They listened—both enthralled and horrified—to stories of brokenness and redemption, pain and loss, joy and despair, and struggles of which they had no idea. Together, we explored the depths of the human condition.

The students began to see medicine not as a collection of science but as a bearer of a certain kind of story and a certain kind of witness. Becoming a physician suddenly meant more than memorizing the Krebs cycle. It meant being present for others. It meant risk, sacrifice, tears, and a raw honesty that most twenty-year-olds aren't truly ready to embrace. Yet embrace it they did, and for that, I am eternally grateful.

As the program grew and students encouraged me to write down the stories, *The Waco Tribune-Herald* agreed to publish a biweekly column on health care. But I didn't want these essays to fall into a "disease of the week" trap, nor did I want them to rail about healthcare economics and reform. I simply wanted to convey to readers the immediateness of the daily life of medicine. Using words to paint pictures of very real situations, I wanted to provoke a conversation on what we as a people want from our healthcare encounters. Words surely fall short of experiences, but words are all we have until we experience the real thing. The stories then were tantalizing tastes and brief glimpses of a system changing before our eyes. They were written for physicians, patients, and anyone who works in the healthcare field—indeed, for all of us.

While the articles were not syndicated, I was surprised to receive emails from all over the country with wonderful and helpful feedback. The column seemed to touch a nerve in readers both within and outside of the medical field who understood what is at stake. You see, the problem really isn't whatever happens to be the hot-button issue of the day. When I talk to patients, colleagues, and readers, we all know intuitively that the real issues run deeper and stem from the heart of our common humanity. We can perhaps avoid the polarizing aspects of the current debates and focus on how we can all learn from a past that is indeed a glimpse into a holy calling.

Of course, all good things must come to an end. After three years, the newspaper was sold to a national media chain, and the new owners wanted nationally syndicated columnists. I received my first—and hopefully last—pink slip. And with it, I gladly transitioned to retirement. Since then, people have asked if I would consider writing a book based on my articles, and in time, I agreed.

Thus, *Medicine at the Crossroads* was born. It is a collection of essays that touches on three perspectives: the physicians, the patients, and the healthcare system. Each essay addresses a pressing question.

While the collection originated in the classroom among scores of bright, inquisitive students, it is intended for all of us. Whether you are a physician, patient, or any other participant in the healthcare system, may you be bold enough, humble enough, and vulnerable enough to listen to these stories—and to the stories of those around you—with wonder and awe.

And while this collection may offer some solutions with "fear and trembling," it does not dare claim to have all the answers. The purpose is simply to start conversations. So, let us all take a collective breath and examine our personal feelings and expectations of medicine. May we each glimpse our own possibilities and discover our own fresh, creative solutions.

Ultimately, *Medicine at the Crossroads* is my stained

glass window for the world. Individually, each story of illness, medicine, and healing provides a tiny, fragmented glimpse into the heart of a problem. Collectively, my hope is that these stories forge together to reveal a larger narrative truth.

Together, let us find our way to compassionate, humane health care for all. Let us find healing—for ourselves, our loved ones, and our system.

Michael Attas

ACKNOWLEDGMENTS

I would like to thank the thousands of Baylor pre-medical students who listened with wonder and awe as I told stories that attempted to shape a certain vision of health care. Their feedback, friendships, and support of both the Medical Humanities Program and me were important as this "way of thinking about medicine" was born and grew into maturity.

In addition, the leadership at Baylor who trusted me with a vision of a Medical Humanities Program was invaluable, as it provided a fertile and receptive audience among bright, young healthcare professionals-to-be. Their willingness to open themselves up to the world of pain, loss, and finally growth shaped the tone and flavors of this project. In particular, Judge Ken Starr arrived at Baylor when the program could very well have sunk under the weight of rapid growth and limited resources. His quiet yet firm support set us on a solid foundation that is still bearing fruit and literally changing the face of health care that our young physicians now practice.

Finally, a huge thank you must go to the former owner, publisher, and editor of the Waco Tribune-Herald: Clifton Robinson, Dan Savage, and Carlos Sanchez, respectively. They gave me the freedom to explore, create, and find my writing voice. That gift shaped my life in ways that words can never truly describe nor measure.

THE PHYSICIAN

"In seeking absolute truth, we aim at the unattainable and must be content with broken portions."

—WILLIAM OSLER

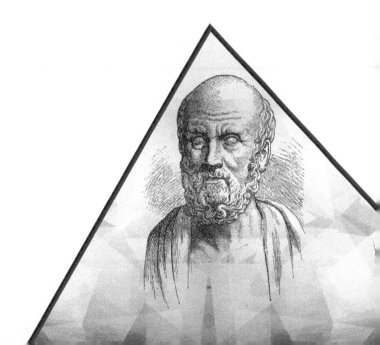

THE PARADOX
OF SERVICE

Is service enough of a reason to be in medicine?

Let me ask you a question: why are you in medicine? When I ask my students this question, I hear all sorts of reasons why they choose this profession. Some, for example, choose it for financial gain. I tell them that if they want to make a lot of money, they're in the wrong building. They need to transfer to the business school. I say this because if they view medicine as only a business, they'll be left adrift when the business model changes, as it inevitably will.

Some choose medicine for pride and prestige. But as far as prestige is concerned, the days are over when physicians and pastors topped the lists of respected jobs. The prestige of health care, at least according to public perception, has plummeted in survey after survey, and often for valid reasons.

Others choose this profession because they are skilled in the sciences and problem-solving. They say they enjoy the intellectual or technical challenge. But humans are more than problems to be solved. We are mysteries to be lived and experienced. We're relational beings with stories and realities and illnesses. In some aspects, we are all broken and wounded. The vulnerability that comes with that is what finally brings a patient to our offices or hospitals. Bearing the gift of trust given us by our patients can be a demanding and daunting task—one that is not fully accomplished by the sciences. Those who view medicine as strictly problem-solving will find themselves at an emotional rock bottom when the science fails.

While we certainly need to excel in our technical skills and business understandings, we must possess a greater motivation to commit to a life in medicine. In spite of these faulty reasons for entering the profession, I would venture that, at some level, most people buy into the notion of service.

But is service enough of a reason to go into medicine?

Even for those of us who are motivated by service, the outcomes are looking bleak. Study after study shows that satisfaction scores are at an all-time low both for patients and providers. Physicians are burning out early and retiring at younger and younger ages. Nurses are in danger of becoming jaded and callous. Rather than embracing radical changes and challenges of the status quo, many of us are fearful. We're plunging headlong toward a major shortage of physicians in this country, and we can ill afford to lose any more of the best and the brightest. If this trend isn't reversed, we are heading off of the cliff in the way we all experience medicine and illness.

To break this decline within our healthcare community, we need to take a closer look at our reasons for going into medicine. In particular, we need to take a closer look at our notion of service.

In a letter to one of the earliest Christian churches, an apostle named Paul used the word "kenosis" to describe service.[1] "Kenosis" may be a single Greek word, but it contains an entirely rich, existential perspective of life. It refers to a "self-emptying" sacrificial love.

In true kenosis, each of us is a vessel full of love that we empty and then refill. It is considered by some as a model for not only human and religious behavior, but for the notion of vocation in certain fields. Indeed, for those in the healing professions, kenosis is the bedrock of our history.

Here is where a paradox occurs: when our vessels of love are emptied, we are refilled again by acts of loving service to others. Kenosis is a continual, unbroken circle of being refilled by first being emptied.

Herein lies a problem in medicine: many healthcare providers resist this true notion of service. They don't allow their vessels to run dry. "Don't get involved in patients' lives," they reason with themselves. "The emotional cost is too high." They focus only on the medical

---

1   *New American Standard Bible* © 1995, Philippians 2:7.

issues, expecting science do its magic. For them, medicine isn't about service; it's about biomedical problem-solving.

But there's a danger in emptying our vessels dry and not filling them back up again—or refilling them with the wrong things. This is partly the reason physicians have higher incidences of suicides, divorces, substance abuse, and depression than the general population. I believe the rejection of kenosis is responsible for the high anxiety among health care professionals.

At this point in history, it is more important than ever to honestly identify our reasons for going into medicine. A primary desire for wealth, prestige, or problem-solving is not enough to bear the demands of medicine. Without an understanding of kenosis, we won't be able to meet our patients' deepest needs. It is only this kind of self-emptying service that will gratify their needs—as well as our own.

SHADES OF GRAY

How can we be certain about life-and-death decisions in a world of uncertainty?

We seem to live in a world of certainty, of black and white. That's why respect for nuanced differences of opinion and civilized discourse is fading at all levels of society—and nowhere is this problem more apparent than in the academic classroom. Students often arrive at medical school with firmly held religious and political beliefs, many of which they've inherited from their parents. They see ambiguity as a weakness; there are no shades of gray in their beliefs.

But in the world of biomedical ethics, human dilemmas are always couched in just such shades. Here, the certainty of youth invariably bumps up against the hard reality of very human problems and patients—like the 16-year-old that arrived in the emergency room where I was on duty.

She was an unwed mother who had delivered a beautiful baby girl, and now she was desperately short of breath. Within twelve hours she was on life support. She had a form of congestive heart failure and was rapidly declining, so in an effort to stave off an almost-certain heart transplant, we installed a heart-assist pump to rest her heart until a suitable donor could be found. But after a few weeks, her heart miraculously began to slowly recover. Eventually she stabilized, went home, and recovered perfectly. She resumed her high school studies and graduated with honors.

But one year later, while a student at college, she became pregnant again, which threatened her life once more. We were left with Solomon's dilemma. On the one hand, carrying the pregnancy to term would almost certainly lead to two deaths: hers and that of her unborn child. Furthermore, no one in her community was willing to take responsibility for her first child, who would be left orphaned. On the other hand, terminating the pregnancy obviously would result in the death of an unborn child while saving the life of the mother, and this option was against her religious beliefs.

Do we sacrifice a life in the name of principles? Who decides? And upon what moral or political or theological basis is that decision to be made?

When I present the case of this young mother to students, it inevitably causes an uproar. Students argue passionately with each other. Some weep at the injustice of reality. All are astounded that physicians have to guide people gently to a place of healing where no "choice" is ideal.

These students are learning that ambiguity is simply an acknowledgment of human frailty, and that medical ethics is not math or rocket science. They're realizing that, more often than not, there truly isn't a right answer. The answers are usually shrouded in mystery and ambiguity, leaving people wounded in its wake. Students who were radically pro-life suddenly realize that choices of life and death are complex, and students who are pro-choice realize the choice itself is costly. And it's only the beginning: in this profession, they will witness the most painful of human choices, and the decisions will never be easy.

Never is a dilemma more intense than when considering euthanasia. I bring this issue to light in the classroom by reading a first-person account published in the *Journal of the American Medical Association* in 1988. It was written by an anonymous intern who was caring for a woman dying of metastatic cancer.

The patient was in horrible, unrelenting pain because the pain relief was not working any longer. She had no more than a few days or weeks to live. One night, in agony and despair, the woman pleaded with the intern, "Let's get this over with."

Out of deep frustration and compassion, the intern brought a terminal dose of narcotics into the room. When her rate of breathing slowed and then ceased, he said, "It's over, Debbie."[2]

These words have become one of the most famous lines in medical ethics literature. While not explicitly saying so, the *Journal of the American Medical Association*

---

2   Name withheld by request, "It's Over, Debbie," *Journal of the American Medical Association*, 1988, as accessed April 25, 2018, at www.mclean.k12.ky.us/docs/Its%20Over%20Debbie.pdf.

made it clear that he had helped the woman end life on her terms.

As expected, the article created a firestorm in medical, legal, and ethical worlds. The case was an example of what is now called active, voluntary euthanasia. It's when a patient in a hopelessly terminal case –and with full, informed consent—simply requests help in dying. It is an active, free choice.

At that time, participating in what is now called physician-assisted suicide was illegal nationwide, as it still is in many states. Many prosecutors promised to bring charges of homicide against the intern if they could discover his identity, which the publication did not reveal. This was before the Kevorkian era, when a handful of pioneering states and ethicists began to present euthanasia and physician-assisted suicide as reasonable choices that people of faith and strong morality could openly discuss. They were talking about death with dignity, though it was not something that many spoke of in public. If it were discussed, the subject was never intended to leave the door open for healthcare professionals to expedite a patient's demise.

But this discussion needs to be placed in the context of other forms of euthanasia. Active, *involuntary* euthanasia, for example, is supported by a majority of Americans when it takes the form of capital punishment in the justice system. Another form that is requested by some terminally ill patients and their families is *passive* euthanasia, which is the withholding of treatment. A respirator, for instance, is disconnected from a braindead patient, and the decision is made to withhold intravenous fluids or antibiotics. Passive euthanasia is about letting nature take its course. In this regard, we could say that euthanasia is a part of every hospital in the country when we consider that most Americans now have "advanced medical directives" that guide healthcare professionals through the ethical quagmire of end-of-life decisions.

Even in the context of these other forms of euthanasia, for many of us there is something still profoundly disturbing about helping a person end life, even when the patient's days are limited. It tugs not only at our emotional heartstrings but also our sense of ethical and religious norms and values. It gets at the heart of what our civilization stands for.

Given all of these profoundly complex issues, how can we be certain about life-and-death decisions in a world of uncertainty?

We can begin by examining the goals and values of our religious traditions and by defining our highest value. I believe that a goal shared by many religious traditions is the relief of suffering based on compassionate love. I would also submit that biological life, while important, can be worshipped to the point of idolatry.

When we insist, for instance, on prolonging life at *all* costs, we seem to be placing our own needs and beliefs above that of our patients'. Preservation of life at the expense of dignity and freedom is often a misguided attempt to deny our patients something they all want: the freedom to choose the terms of their passing from this world. Extending the life of a person whose suffering is agonizing seems almost inhumane and narcissistic of us as healers; we often treat our pets with more dignity and compassion.

While I may not know the best answer to such medical ethical issues, I believe euthanasia is an act that can indeed be performed out of profound love and respect for human life and dignity. For me, it is consistent with my own religious tradition and faith, though others may vehemently disagree.

Which brings me to my next point: as we grapple with these profound dilemmas, we must not leave these conversations solely to politicians, protesters, or academic ethicists. We should strive to discuss our opinions with each other with respect and civility. Our classrooms should be the places where young adults can explore their belief systems and work out their understanding of complex issues.

And more than anything, we must accept that this world is never as simple as it seems. Because until you have had a dying young woman weep in your arms about the choices she faces, you cannot begin to imagine the complexity of those decisions. It is only with this humble perspective that we can gently walk our patients into those dark places, providing non-judgmental love, light, and hope in a world of pain.

IF YOU WERE ME

What would you do if you were me?

"What would you do if you were me?"

It's a question that I am repeatedly asked by patients. On the surface, it's a pretty simple, straightforward request. It really doesn't demand much except an honest opinion.

Yet this question gets at the heart of medical ethics. These patients are really asking about two of the four classic principles in medical ethics: *non-malfeasance* and *beneficence*. Non-malfeasance means "do no harm," and beneficence means "do good." They are simple guides that have been foundational for medicine and the healing arts since the time of Hippocrates. As physicians, we like to think that these two pillars are still the foundations of our decisions. And as patients, we rightly expect them to be. We all know intuitively that these mandates should be at the heart of every healthcare encounter.

Yet non-malfeasance and beneficence are increasingly difficult to implement in the current healthcare environment. I submit that, for a myriad of reasons, we are losing these ethical norms by the day. Health care is becoming a runaway locomotive.

Case in point: the system is increasingly driven by technology, pharmaceuticals, hospital competition, and physician preferences. Mergers and acquisitions, previously limited to the world of high finance, are becoming the norm and not the exception in the world of health care. Young physicians emerging from their training with mountains of debt no longer have the luxury of joining small groups of like-minded colleagues. More than likely they will sell their services to the highest bidder. But this is a Faustian bargain that puts their long-term satisfaction and joy in peril.

Consider also the introduction of a new technology or drug. When it is compared invariably to older modalities, often the simple message is "newer and better." Yet to bring that technology or drug to market, a company is only required to demonstrate that it isn't any worse than what is already available. Perfectly good procedures, drugs, and equipment are replaced with newer generations of products that aren't always better or safer.

This leads to another issue: the cost of a new technology or drug almost always winds up being more expensive, even if it isn't any better than the old one. Of course, the consumer bears the burden of that cost through higher premiums and higher costs, many of which duplicate what is already available. This reveals one of the surprising things about healthcare economics, which is that an explosion of competition and technology doesn't result in the lowering of costs; it invariably raises them. Health care doesn't follow normal market supply-and-demand curves.

Amid all of these issues, the fact is that most patients and families want the best technology. And physicians want their patients to have the best. In our drive to increase our market share and provide expanded services, how do physicians respond when patients ask:

"What would you do if you were me?"

Let us start by looking more critically at the larger picture. In our zeal to heal, perhaps physicians need to be more aware of the forces that are pushing us in a direction in which we may not always be comfortable. We should resist the sort of mental laziness that allows ourselves to be swayed by market pressures and to make decisions we may come to later regret.

Then let us look critically at these new toys and opportunities. As physicians and other healthcare providers, we must be intellectually honest with ourselves about the risks that go up with the rewards. Yes, we have the ability to do truly miraculous things in medicine, but there is never a free lunch. As technology and procedures become increasingly complex, the risk often escalates exponentially. Many times, the few lives we save with aggressive modalities are counterbalanced by the loss of lives or complications in others by the very same technology. We are at a time in the history of health care when we should be asking ourselves the fundamental question, "Will this procedure help or hurt the patient?"

We must also be bluntly honest with our patients about this fundamental reality. This is not simply a matter of adequately informed consent. This is about being bold enough to simply say when necessary, "We shouldn't be doing this."

Together, we must remember the two commandments: Don't hurt people. Help them. Let us cling to these roots of medicine that are our heart and soul.

A PERSONAL QUESTION

How can physicians change in response to new understandings of faith and spirituality in medicine?

It's inevitable. In the classroom, when I introduce the idea of inquiring into a patient's spirituality, a student almost always pushes back.

"Isn't that, you know, sort of private? Isn't faith a personal question?" asked one young man. He was voicing what some of the others were thinking.

"Well, of course it is," I responded. "But so are bowel movements and sexual habits, and yet we feel free to ask people about them for the sake of good medicine."

It's no wonder the topic of faith seems off-limits and irrelevant. In the medical profession, we have been trained to see our souls and bodies as separate entities.

In 1910, a study called *The Flexner Report*[3] changed American medicine. It was intended to bring medical education into the 20th century by standardizing sciences as the foundation of medicine. A standard curriculum

---

3   Alexander Flexner, *Medical Education in the United States and Canada: A Report to The Carnegie Foundation for the Advancement of Teaching,* (New York: Carnegie Foundation, 1910).

for medical schools was implemented and became the norm in America. Yet nowhere in that curriculum was there room for the idea that a patient's religious beliefs or traditions had a role in wellness.

But practice tells me otherwise. I still remember the first time I clearly saw a distinct relationship between faith and physical wellness. It was thirty years ago, and I entered a clinic room to find an old couple waiting for me. They were stooped and frail, having run a family farm for their entire lives. They were now entering the homestretch, which should have been a rewarding time of rest for them.

But I sensed it was anything but peaceful. The old man had a major heart issue, but this was not what was on their minds that day. It turned out that this couple was in the middle of a major life crisis.

They began to tell me what truly weighed on their souls: they were in deep agony for their son. This was during the early days of the AIDS crisis, and they had just learned that their beloved and only son was dying from the disease. On top of that, they were also struggling with the newfound knowledge that their son was gay. It was just too much for them to get their heads around.

During our subsequent visits, we talked honestly together about big issues like forgiveness and tolerance. We talked about dignity, justice, and healing. In time, they began to see their son as a beloved child of God. And they began to deal honestly with the issues of his disease and impending death. Instead of asking themselves *why*, they began to see that the power of their religious beliefs was their way out of the darkness.

But the most striking thing to me was the impact of their faith on their physical health. They had mistakenly assumed that the father's heart condition and their son's crisis were unrelated, but with each visit, as both parents found peace in their beliefs, they seemed to grow younger and healthier before my eyes. Sure enough, the old man's heart disease had indeed diminished.

This couple had provided great insight to me on the role of faith in the process of disease in patients. Unfortunately, the medical profession would wait nearly another century after *The Flexner Report* to officially recognize this link. It wasn't until the 1990s that the World Health Organization finally added the term "spiritual" to its definition of health, alongside "biological," "sociological," and "psychological."

At about the same time, the idea began to emerge in practice. Leading medical schools such as Duke and George Washington University began to add spirituality to the list of aspects that young students should consider when learning about their patients. And then the Robert Wood Johnson Foundation funded an exploration by six medical schools on the notion of spirituality at the bedside. From that original small group, there are now more than one hundred American medical schools that offer courses in spirituality and health care.

Today, studies affirm that spirituality and faith exert a powerful healing influence. This newer and wiser science views our souls and bodies as two expressions of one divine reality. And when I think back to that couple all those years ago who first proved to me that our spiritual and biological lives are intimately connected, I agree with the new science.

But in the classroom, the question remains: "Isn't this, you know, private?" Even with studies and new evidence that point out the benefit of incorporating a spiritual inventory in the clinical encounter, reluctance still lingers in medicine.

So how can we change in response to new understandings of faith and spirituality in medicine?

Let's start with our education. Medical education at its best should include a cursory overview of all religious traditions. This means religions such as Judaism, Christianity, Islam, Hinduism, Native American spirituality, and others. Only with a respectful understanding of a patient's belief system can we fully engage them as caring providers in a system that is often fragmented.

We are increasingly becoming a culture in which many people are simply not religious in the traditional sense of the word. They may be agnostic or atheistic. These beliefs must be honored and considered with every bit of caring and non-judgmental action as any other belief system.

Let's also address our own timidity when it comes to asking a patient about faith or spirituality. This begins with an understanding that we cannot be complete physicians without listening to the importance of the spiritual beliefs of our patients. To do otherwise is like examining only the right half of the body and ignoring the left half. Faith, including daily habits related to faith, is one critical part of the whole patient.

It is only with this understanding that we can boldly ask our patients about their prayer patterns and the role of faith and community in their lives. And we can ask them in the same simple, direct, non-judgmental way that we ask about their cholesterol and exercise habits. Because, ultimately, these matters of faith have every bit as much to do with health as the physical matters.

Of course, we should continually exercise good judgment here. During a medical illness or life-threatening crisis, for example, is not an appropriate time to attempt to witness to someone. Most Christian patients would not mind a Christian physician witnessing to them, but they would not want a Muslim physician attempting to convert them on their deathbed. Even among Christians, we need to honor denominational differences within their faith, as not all welcome an "intruder" into their spiritual space. We should temper our boldness with respect for the patient and circumstances.

Finally, let's dismantle the idea that prayer is a breach of our relationships with our patients. There is a growing awareness that it makes no more sense for the clinician to ignore the spiritual dimension of our patients' lives than it would be to examine only half of the body. Yes, to be sure, prayer does venture into somewhat unchartered territory between our faith and our patients' faiths.

But it is *not* a breach—quite the contrary. Prayer may be considered a fundamental part of healing for many patients of faith, especially because many patients are wounded or feel vulnerable in healthcare encounters. It is often transformative for the one praying.

Of course, prayer may not be the only conduit towards a healing encounter; additionally, everyone responds differently to the suggestion. Some physicians simply do not want to pray for or with their patients, and even if they do, many patients may be offended by offers of prayers or insistence of prayers at the bedside. Others wholeheartedly welcome the opportunity. One physician I know prays at the patient's bedside for *every* condition, from a diagnosis of colon cancer to poison ivy. In my humble perspective, this is a bit over the top of both utilization and expectations of prayer in the role of health care. I personally think I'd rather save prayer for the big guns and leave the daily sniffles to us humans to sort through, but there certainly may be others who disagree. Wise physicians should remain sensitive to the needs of patients in all situations.

As one trained in both the sciences and theology, I recognize the struggle to find the balance between understanding the faith of our patients and expressing our own authentic beliefs. Persevere in your care for your patients. When in doubt, I personally believe that our faith is *best* witnessed when we leave doctrine to others and focus on practicing sound, compassionate medicine. I've read that St. Francis once said, "Preach always; only when necessary use words."

WINTER OF GRACE

How can we help families adapt to a radically changed person in their lives?

"Would you tell Dad he can't drive anymore?"

I looked at grown children standing before me. This family was negotiating illness leading to death. In their struggle to manage their expectations and emotions, they were drawing me, as their physician, into an intimate part of their relationships.

I looked at their elderly father. Inevitably, some of his faculties and abilities had diminished. It happens at a different rate for every one of us. Some patients in their 80s or even 90s still have wonderful vision, hearing, and reflexes. Some in their 50s find their bodies already betraying them, and they simply cannot cope with the demands of autonomous living. Others see their truest and best selves become diminished or lost by disease.

This entire period of life is different for each of us. I often see that patients who live good and harmonious lives enter this stage peacefully. It becomes a "winter grace," as Dr. Kathleen Fischer called it in her book,

Winter Grace: Spirituality and Aging.[4] In my experience, it is one of the most sacred periods of our lives. Some of my patients age so gracefully and powerfully that they become beacons of light and hope for everyone they encounter. They love without reservation and have an innate wisdom that draws people like a magnet to them.

Others rage against the dying of the light, as in Dylan Thomas' poem to his father, "Do Not Go Gentle Into that Good Night."[5] These are often the patients who have struggled with life, and they enter this stage with difficulty. Their lives are constant sorrow, anger, and frustration about the passage of time and the toll it takes on the human condition.

Whether this is a season of grace or sorrow seems to center on how we regard the memories of our lives. Our memories are not simply fossilized reflections on a distant past that no longer exists; Presbyterian minister and author Frederick Buechner thinks they are an important way we can continue to learn and grow in our later years. Memories become a lived reality that continues to shape the world around us. We reach into the past to allow us to move into the mystery of the future. How well we do this determines how well we move into the winter of our lives with dignity and freedom.

But even the most dignified patients may see great transformation when it comes to disease. When people

---

4   Kathleen Fischer, *Winter Grace: Spirituality and Aging,* (Tennessee: Upper Room, 1998).

5   Dylan Thomas, "Do Not Go Gentle Into the Good Night," *In Country Sleep.* (New York: New Directions, 1952).

who have lived all of their lives in a state of health move to a state of disease, they are changed. Sometimes illness brings out the best in them. They become more tolerant of themselves and others. Rigidity is replaced with flexibility, and sternness with a wry sense of humor.

Yet reality is a cruel mistress, and illness may rob them of everything they hold to be true. When this happens, their emotional, spiritual, and practical resources are strained to the breaking point. They find that they are human after all, and they struggle with great issues that can overwhelm the strongest and most dedicated among us. Sometimes, in this painful change, illness creates an almost impenetrable layer surrounding their core identities. Their kindness is replaced with rage; compassion and tolerance are replaced with a short fuse; wisdom with adolescence.

The changes that come from illness often make the patient seem like a stranger to those who know them well. Family members are left confused about the new person in their midst; indeed, physicians can face intense encounters with patients who have changed because of an illness. While all of us recognize that Alzheimer's disease can alter a patient's personality, in my experience, any profound illness can result in similar changes. "What has happened to my spouse or parent?" their families ask. The person standing before them isn't the same as the one they've known and loved for forty years.

To add to this confusion, we live in a society that is increasingly fragmented and mobile. Practical considerations must be acknowledged. *Where are we going to live?*

*How are we going to get from point A to point B? How do
we manage our finances?*

All of these issues are tangible and visible reminders to the elderly of the realities they do not want to face. That is why, as I looked at my elderly patient and his family standing before me, I knew their question was more significant than a set of keys. It was highly symbolic of an agonizing struggle about freedom and autonomy that was being met with fierce resistance. And as their physician, they wanted me to be the enforcer. However, the healthcare system is ill-equipped to help people understand how difficult it can be for patients and families to find a total stranger in their midst.

How can we help families adapt to a radically changed person in their lives?

There are a few things we can do for them. First, we can help them to recognize the process of disease. Disease is best seen as a temporary interruption in the journey from the "kingdom of disease" back to the "kingdom of health," as one writer describes it. This is a journey back to wholeness and restoration. Sometimes diseases can be conquered, and the journey from brokenness to wholeness becomes a path of self-discovery.

We can also help them by recognizing the toll of disease. We should acknowledge that the painful realities of disease and illness place an external layer over the true self, masking the inner self from their loved ones. They need reassurance that the truest self of their loved one, the one created by God at the very core of their existence, has not been destroyed. It is still there, very deep inside. The goodness is still there, and it may occasionally peek through in the simplest of ways.

Physicians need to be conversant in the demands that illness can impose on patients and families, and at the barest minimum help patients and their families seek out appropriate resources. This includes strongly encouraging that caregivers seek out others who have traveled the same road. They need to find support groups and seek wise counsel—as do we.

Finally, we as caregivers need time to restore ourselves. We need to engage in solitude that renews; we need a community that heals; we need relationships grounded in love. All of these are restorative lifelines for a journey that we all must travel.

I've found these discussions with families to be daunting. As we grapple with the mortality of a loved one, we are provided glimpses of our own mortality. But these conversations can also be liberating—if they are based upon love, respect, and the dignity of the patient. When we honor a life well lived, we can find common ground between the health and well-being of our patients and the larger needs of our society.

A MORAL CLAIM

Is honesty always the best policy?

It took me years to get over the first death of a patient during my internship. At first, I was distraught—a feeling that I passed off for a while as the typical loss one feels as a young physician. Yet it persisted. I had this gnawing feeling that I somehow should have done more. And so, when I found myself still dreaming about this man after several years, I knew something was wrong.

The patient I had treated was a wonderful tobacco farmer from the Appalachians who had widespread pancreatic cancer. His illness was beyond treatment, and his decline was swift. In the brief time that I had with him, I was afforded beautiful glimpses into his life. I appreciated the dignity and calmness he showed in his final days.

I knew all along that his disease was terminal, and the patient faced the end of his life with grace. Why then, despite these facts, did I feel that I had failed him?

I've learned that our interactions with patients often uncover issues in our inner lives that need attention, and it would be years before I finally uncovered the problem: I had not spoken the truth that he needed to hear.

He knew he was dying. He was at peace with that knowledge. I knew he was dying, too. Yet I hid behind a mass of statistics and medical jargon. I did what I was trained to do: I presented his options with formality, objectivity, and sterility, and then I let him decide.

Sure, patients deserve to be at the center of their medical decision-making. This is called patient autonomy, and it is a bedrock in biomedical ethics. Perhaps rightly so. But it took me years to learn that patients also want to know what their physicians *think*. They want us to simply sit down with them and discuss their plans for death.

This stark perspective was engrained in me about 15 years ago, when I visited Dr. Ed Pellegrino, the professor of Medical Ethics at Georgetown Medical School at the time. He is considered the leading Christian medical ethicist of our time. My hope was to wade with him into deeply complex and nuanced ethical debates about issues such as euthanasia, right to life, and nutritional support.

But Dr. Pellegrino had other ideas. As I followed him on his rounds, I observed the physician talking to patients about their lives, their loves, and their losses. He was talking to his staff about how they were handling certain issues. He was leading them gently—as all good teachers do—toward a more holistic approach to medicine, one that didn't stop at charts and statistics but that ventured into mystery and even grace.

One day during rounds together, he motioned me

into a break room and said something that would change my life. "Mike," he told me, "remember that our patients have a moral claim on our lives."

Most physicians would balk at the implication of that claim. We tend to be rugged individualists, and it might go against our grain to accept that patients have a claim on us.

But it's a profound truth. We exist not in isolation, but as a part of something larger than ourselves. The poet John Donne said it best: "No man is an island, entire of itself; every man is a piece of the continent, a part of the main."[6]

Patients want us to simply speak the truth in language they can understand. They want to know what our experience tells us about their illness and what lies ahead. They want honesty, not ambiguity. They want clarity, not data. Often they will ask, "What would you do if you were me?" The answer to this question has become my litmus test of any decision.

But is honesty always the best policy?

Even with the best intentions, the issue of honesty and clarity can be blurry. The decision to be honest may lead to conflict and poor outcomes, as I learned in the case of a bright, 80-year-old woman who was diagnosed with a form of bone cancer.

---

6   John Donne, "Meditation XVII: No Man is an Island," *Devotions upon Emergent Occasions*, (England, 1624).

Before falling ill, the patient had earned a reputation in a large corporation as an administrative assistant who clearly ran the whole show, so there was no reason to believe she wouldn't be fully in charge of her medical treatment as well. By the time I began to see her, she had already begun extensive chemotherapy, and she was approaching everything we threw at her with an upbeat and optimistic demeanor.

Yet the reports from her oncologist were not encouraging. I began to feel a bit disconnected from her disease and its implications in my role as her cardiologist, so I called the specialist to ask about her disease and its prognosis. The oncologist told me the patient had less than six months to live.

"Have you told her?" I asked him.

"No, of course not," he said. "I don't think she's ready to hear that news."

But I was convinced that this patient knew her time was nearing its end, just as the tobacco farmer had known. This woman remained a warm, interesting, and loving person, yet my intuition told me that she had come to terms with her mortality.

At her next appointment with me, she brought her two grown children. When I had a chance to speak with both of them outside the room about their mother's prognosis, I asked whether or not she had been told the truth.

"No," her daughter said. "We don't want Mom to know the truth. It would kill her."

Her son strongly disagreed. "I think Mom has a right to know and to make plans for the end of her life."

What is a physician to do in a case like this? Temper the truth-telling to keep families together and to protect the emotional state of the patient? Or be frank about a dismal prognosis because the patient deserves to be informed and to make informed decisions?

The American Medical Association's panel on biomedical ethics is clear on the issue. It says that the cornerstone of any decision-making is patient autonomy, which states the obvious: the patient should always remain at the center of decisions. Our moral contract is with the patient, not the children or spouses.

But reality isn't always as clear. Studies show that patients tend to hear what they want. Some want hope; others want unvarnished truth. And in the case of this patient, the issue is further muddled when others are involved. This disagreement had already shattered the family unity, and the resulting stress engulfed all of us on the medical team as well. The patient was caught in the middle.

Unfortunately, such fractured situations are becoming increasingly common in a healthcare system with increasingly fragmented care. Patients and their families are coping with these difficult decisions with multiple specialists and primary care physicians. We often face the impossible choices of giving patients hope, telling some hard truths, or appeasing family who are at odds about what to do. It's a delicate balancing act that involves artistry and agony, far from the comforting absolutism of science. It leaves us groping our way with through the murky, gray area of diplomacy.

To make matters worse, these choices are influenced by the federal government and private insurers. It's astounding that both are willing to pay exorbitant fees for technical end-of-life procedures that are neither medically advisable nor proven effective, yet neither is willing to spend money for something as simple as time for a physician to discuss end-of-life issues with a patient.

Take, for instance, a heart defibrillator as an end-of-life treatment. We can implant this technology even though we often have no data that it will prolong life for many subsets of people with heart disease. Yet when we do, we're reimbursed handsomely by the insurer and government. Almost twenty percent of our federal health dollars are spent on end-of-life treatments with futile outcomes like a heart defibrillator.

Now compare this to the ten or twenty hours we spend with patients and families in their time of greatest need. Personally, I find this time with patients among my most emotionally and spiritually rewarding. However, the powers that be have decided that it is without economic value and, therefore, without any value at all. There is no "billable code" for this time, which means it is essentially donated. As a society, we value technology over wisdom; we value procedures over guidance. As a result, our patients are often left in the dark when they need us the most.

Because of the raging debate among healthcare experts over the disproportionate reimbursement for procedures as opposed to cognitive input and time, there is a trend in medicine to finally begin to pay for cognitive skills and not just procedural skills. But even this progress brings its problems: some claim that this will result in death panels. This is political demagoguery, plain and simple. When politicians resort to this sort of insult to the medical profession, it is obvious that they have not had a loved one in these situations.

Amid all of these fragments and disagreements, let us as physicians bring honesty and clarity to the system. We can do this by creating a loving, supportive system that encourages all providers to have honest and realistic discussions. This means creating a system that reimburses us fairly and respectfully for end-of-life issues.

And let us bring honesty and clarity to our patients by finding a way to validate important conversations. We must resist a cold recitation of the facts and rushing to the next exam room, which tends to bring even more pain and frustration to patients. In his classic book, *Anatomy of Hope*, Dr. Jerome Groopman gives pointers on how to have these conversations. He says that talking about the grimmest of situations in hopeful terms is often the wisest and kindest thing we can do for our patients. He doesn't recommend glossing over the truth, but he does recommend telling it in language that leaves opens the door for hope, a strong variable that can positively improve many forms of treatment. We honor our patients by having these kinds of conversations.

I had the opportunity to provide this kind of honor to a rancher for whom I had cared for nearly twenty years who had rapidly advancing heart disease. I had come to know him and his family quite well, and after repeated hospitalizations for congestive heart failure, he was running out of options. All he wanted to do was go home to watch his momma cows and their babies playing in the bluebonnets of a Texas spring one more time. His land, his cattle, and his family had defined his life, and he wanted to die in their presence.

So, along with his wife and children, we began to have conversations about his future and his options. They were no-nonsense kind of folks, so they welcomed the direct, to-the-point discussions that were both necessary and heartbreaking. We talked about home health hospice, do-not-resuscitate status, life support systems, and approaches to end-of-life decisions. They found relief in our honest, compassionate dialogue. And of course, as if grace had emerged from our shared conversations, he indeed lived until the spring welcomed both his bluebonnets and his calves. And then he died, surrounded by the love of his family in his land that he cherished.

Years later, I was allowed the same opportunity with my own mother. Like the rancher, she needed help to sort through end-of-life issues, but her own physician didn't take the time to have such dialogue. I didn't like having these conversations that were honest and painful. But this is where medicine becomes more than science; it becomes an art. As she approached the end of her time, our conversations became healing. Ultimately, my mother died with respect and dignity. She deserved nothing less.

LESSONS FROM A DEATHBED

How can physicians help patients and their family members cope with moments of crisis in the hospital setting?

It was one of the hardest days of my medical career. A 20-year-old college student on a respirator in the intensive care unit had been pronounced braindead.

There had been discussions with the family about organ donation. There had been the question of "why" this illness. There had been the many other questions that had no answers. Finally, the decision was made to disconnect his life support.

No one was exempt from the pain of this tragedy. Tears flowed from nurses, staff, family, friends, and roommates as we gathered around the bedside to prepare for his passing.

There are two aspects of this moment that are worth deeper reflection.

One aspect is the room in which we gathered. In modern American medicine, death almost always occurs in a hospital setting such as the one in which we stood. This is a remarkable change from a century ago, when most deaths came at home.

Another aspect is the people who gathered around the young man as he passed. A century ago, he would have been in the presence of family and loved ones. But today, the death of a patient most often occurs surrounded by strangers. The primary care physician—who knows the patient best—rarely comes to the hospital any more. The specialists are not privy to the nuances of the family's emotional and spiritual needs. Often, only the nurses provide an anchor for a dying patient, as they are there for long shifts while physicians come and go.

Patients are dying in strange rooms among strangers. Many times, healthcare encounters are sterile and void of meaning.

How can we help patients and their family members cope with moments of crisis in hospitals?

One way to help is through symbols and rituals. Humans have known for eons that symbolic acts provide closure and allow a sort of healing to occur in the midst of tragedy. Carl Jung, the pioneer in analytical psychology, concluded that symbols and rituals are among the most *powerful* things humans can provide for each other. Yet the truth is that, in medicine, we have not tapped into this power to help patients and families navigate crisis. Hospitals, by their very nature, simply haven't been designed to provide this kind of help.

While it may not be reasonable to expect all physicians to participate in bedside rituals, we all need to be aware of their power. We can give ourselves the freedom to imagine new ways that help patients and families navigate crisis. We can develop a ritual for various healthcare encounters such as death, birth, and life-threatening surgeries.

In addition to rituals, another way to help is to give patients permission to die. This may come as some surprise, given that patients often seem to know when it is time to go. In fact, I've learned from my experience in the ICU that patients are often the *first* to know when it is time to go. Our bodies have wisdom that is beyond intellectual knowledge and brain activity. But even with this intuition, patients sometimes still need permission. They need to be told by family or staff or clergy that it is alright to let go of the struggle. I've seen patients choose to die on their own terms, waiting for an event such as a grandchild's wedding or a soldier's safe return home to surrender their spirit and pass on. Given permission and rituals, they can end their journeys with a sense of peace.

Perhaps it was this innate yearning for peace that prompted us to spontaneously reach for each other around the bed of the young college student lying brain-dead before us. A circle of loved ones and strangers held hands and, while the monitor beeped steady and strong, we recited Psalm 23.[7]

> The LORD is my shepherd,
> I shall not want.
> He makes me lie down in green pastures;
> He leads me beside quiet waters.
> He restores my soul;
> He guides me in the paths of righteousness
> For His name's sake.

As we said the words, his heart rate began to slowly decline. These sacred words that we were sharing in the last moments of his life were a visible and concrete ritual.

> Even though I walk through the valley of the shadow of death,
> I fear no evil, for You are with me;
> Your rod and Your staff, they comfort me.
> You prepare a table before me in the presence of my enemies;
> You have anointed my head with oil;
> My cup overflows.
> Surely goodness and lovingkindness will follow me all the days of my life,
> And I will dwell in the house of the LORD forever.

---

7   *New American Standard Bible* © 1995, Psalm 23.

As we quietly finished the last words, the monitor flatlined. He was gone. In that moment of stillness and deep loss, we were enveloped in grace.

AT A LOSS FOR WORDS

What should physicians say to patients in their times of grief?

My first act as an ordained minister was to preach at the funeral of a young man. He wasn't just any young man. He was the son of a close friend. I had held him as an infant, and he had been named after me. Now, twenty-eight years later, he was a graduate student in molecular biology who was found dead in his apartment. He died of an allergic reaction to a prescription arthritis medication. I had just finished my theological education and was still immersed in the real world of clinical medicine, but I realized quickly how unprepared I was for the task.

His parents and I experienced a grief unlike any I had ever known. We had each lost parents, but that seemed part of the natural cycle of life and death. The senselessness and injustice of the death of this young adult was not part of the understandable cycle. Children are not supposed to die before their parents. This harsh reality takes its toll on survivors: studies have shown that parents who have lost children have much higher than normal incidences of divorce, depression, and even suicide.

Yale Divinity School professor Nicholas Wolterstorff wrote about this unbearable grief in a book called *Lament for a Son*. When his son died in a mountain-climbing accident, he didn't sugarcoat his rage, his questions to God, or his sense of alienation and suffering. "Death is the great leveler, so our writers have always told us. Of course, they are right," he said. "But they have neglected to mention the uniqueness of each death and the solitude of suffering which accompanies that uniqueness. I know how you are feeling, we hear. But they don't."[8]

No amount of language, theology, or intimacy can prepare us for the kind of suffering that can devastate the strongest of humans. Physicians often stand at the crossroads of this suffering. In medical school, they don't teach you what to say or how to act when a patient or friend relates what has happened. This is why physicians tend to leave the task of comforting grieving patients to other professionals: pastors, rabbis, and grief counselors. But there are a few simple things we can say that may provide a foothold for grieving patients.

What should physicians say to patients in their times of grief?

Let's take cues from Wolterstorff and start with what

8   Nicholas Wolterstorff, *Lament for a Son*, (Michigan: William B. Eerdmans Publishing Company, 1987).

not to say. Do not prescribe medication unnecessarily. Do not gloss it over. And do not sugarcoat their grief with pious platitudes. I've heard words at the bedside to the effect of, "Well, God just needed your son with him in heaven." For one thing, I don't feel that God causes human suffering so much as he allows it as a part of our freedom; it is an inescapable part of our destiny. For another, these words rarely provide the comfort they were intended to bring. To the contrary, these well-meaning words can cut deep and further wound suffering parents.

Instead, let us begin by acknowledging the suffering of our patients. Like any wise spiritual leader, let them know you are aware of their burden and that you respect their pain. The reality is that there is a hole in their lives that will never be filled, and to presume otherwise is folly. A simple honoring of this gaping absence is the first step on a lifelong journey for the patient, family, and friends.

Let us then provide permission for our patients to explore their wounds and suffering and the impact on their bodies and spirits. When patients are given the freedom to express their anger, doubts, and grief, then the real healing can begin. We should learn not to take these words personally, even when they result in physical rage—and yes, I, like many other in my field, have been struck, embraced, threatened, and intimidated by grieving family members. It's all in the job description. Moment by moment, day by day, tear after tear, people can begin to heal with our permission.

Finally, encourage patients to surround themselves with those who care enough to embrace, not deny, their suffering. Community is more than a concept or a doctrine; it becomes the fabric of human continuity that will allow life to finally flow back into their broken bodies and souls. As physicians, we join their community the moment we step out of our comfort zones as scientists and move deeply into our own humanity and fears. To me, this is the most holy and honored place we may have with a patient or friend, making their pain—and ours—bearable.

THE OTHER SIDE OF
THE DIVIDE

What is the most meaningful thing a physician can provide during times of unexpected grief?

Several years ago, I was on a ski vacation with six friends. We were all laughing, the issues in our daily lives seeming remote as we enjoyed the brilliant Colorado air and snow. But our wonderful vacation would quickly become a devastating nightmare.

As we made our way down one of the mountains, one of my friends simply collapsed. At first, we thought she had suffered a simple ski injury. But within seconds, it was obvious that a catastrophe had occurred. She was unconscious and without a pulse. The ski patrol arrived within seconds and tried to resuscitate her. She was taken to a local hospital, where my identity was no longer a physician. I became just another person in a strange emergency department, waiting on a loved one in crisis. This was out of my element. I was used to being on the other side of the divide—the chasm that exists often between the physician and the patient.

We all held each other as we waited. We prayed. We wept. We questioned, and we expressed our fears. Two hours later, we were told by a very caring physician that our friend had suffered a spontaneous rupture of a brain aneurysm. Had she been in a large, metro, high-tech hospital when it burst suddenly, the fatal outcome would have been the same.

She was flown to the medical school in Denver where, after forty-eight hours on life support, she was declared dead. Her organs were donated, and her family began their journey back to Texas. They prepared for a funeral that was not part of anyone's wildest imagination just four days earlier.

And in the midst of it all, I was reminded of the fragility of life. We know that life is tenuous. It is a daily gift. But I was—and always will be—astounded at how it can change in a heartbeat. At least with chronic diseases, though also insidious, patients and families are given time to process, question, make decisions, and get their hearts around difficult issues. But a sudden tragedy like my friend's death is almost incomprehensible. It swoops in without warning and flips our worlds upside down. And when it does, it leaves us in a morass of confusion, anger, and heartbreak.

This is what happened to me and my friends in that hospital in Colorado. We were suddenly thrust from the "kingdom of living" to the "kingdom of dying," without being given time to prepare. It was a totally helpless, devastating, and terrifying journey.

Perhaps most terrifying was that I was experiencing it from a side that I was not used to. I was used to working for hours to save the lives of patients I do not know. I was used to searching for difficult words to say to people who were in shock. Unfortunately, I was used to the wrenching pain of loss in those situations, even when the faces were new.

But I was not used to *this*. I was not used to experiencing this pain and shock from the perspective of the patient's family. I suddenly found myself shifting roles from that of a physician to that of a friend and loved one. I experienced firsthand how emotions play out with more intensity and consistency in the emergency room than anywhere—then overcome us in everyday life as well.

I had the same questions as everyone else: "What happened? How can this be? Is there any hope? What should we do?" We are asked these questions thousands of times in our lives as physicians. But to be the one asking the questions . . . this placed me directly in the trenches of pain, death, and loss.

Even now, years later, the nightmare in that Colorado hospital is still a blur. It remains a surreal scene that feels like an eternity ago. I do not clearly remember what I said, either medically or in the prayers that we shared. But there is *one* thing I do remember clearly about the physician attending my friend. I remember not his scientific knowledge, but his kindness and the years of wisdom he shared.

What is the most meaningful thing a physician can provide during times of unexpected grief?

The physician was not immune to the pain, but he focused intensely on his duties. When he came to ask medical questions and, later, to deliver the tragic news, I sensed the caring in his eyes. And this is the one thing that remains vivid in my mind: it was his presence.

Presence. One writer said presence is the holiest thing we can provide for one another in times of suffering. And from my devastating perspective from the other side of the divide, I have to agree.

As healers, we must be fully present to those in need. We don't have to speak words. We don't have to have an answer when there is none. We don't have to reach for the prescription pad or order a test. But we can listen, love, and be still in the midst of the pain. We can give our friends and patients the freedom to grieve fully, to explore the depths of their pain, and to respond with simple care and kindness.

This comes with it the uncomfortable acknowledgement that we are helpless when life changes in a heartbeat. It is a difficult reality for all of us, particularly for physicians because we like to think that we can fix everything. But, while the truth is painful, it may be one of the most important things we accept.

This also comes with it the realization that we must continue to focus on our work, actions, and words. Our body language must somehow convey a gentle presence, love, forgiveness, and shared sorrow. Because, ultimately, it may not be as important as what we say or do. It may be more about being willing to go through the pain with each other. At the end of the day, perhaps the most important thing is that we are simply *there*.

THE FIRST LOSS

Should we allow ourselves the risk of loving and caring for patients?

I remember my first loss like it was yesterday. She may not have been the first patient I had watched die, but she was the first to whom I'd been personally attached.

She was the wife of the dean of the dental school, a very beautiful and loving woman with a tremendous family. My wife and I had moved to an adjacent farm and became close to not only her and her husband but also their son and daughter-in-law, whose children were born within weeks of our own children. We became so close that we considered one another extended family.

And I? Well, at the time, I was an intern and was, like some interns, a combination of insufferable cockiness and arrogance. Of course, these were just masks to hide the fact that I was scared out of my wits most of the time. I knew a lot of facts but had not yet had *real* live human beings depend upon me for life and death and wisdom. I was firmly entrenched in the model of medical education at the time, and the mantra was simple: learn the facts, practice good medicine, detach from the outcome, and move on to the next patient. And yet, in my arrogance and naiveté, I was about to break every rule in the book.

We were enjoying the friendship of our neighbors when we learned that the dean's wife had a rare and fatal form of heart disease. We all knew her time was limited. It was unfair and devastating, and we were heartbroken. Nonetheless, we soldiered on, sharing bread together during long, lovely meals. We filled our time with wine, food, and one another's company, laughing and telling stories, praying and sometimes weeping. All the while, we awaited the inevitable to happen. And it did.

Six months after her diagnosis, my dear friend, the wife of the dean, died as we knew she would.

I felt like a failure. I felt that I had let her and her whole family down. I was bereft, drowning in self-pity and regrets. I had a sense that I simply was not prepared for this life in medicine, with its ongoing loss and pain. I wanted to quit. As if the pain wasn't unbearable enough, my chief of cardiology expected me to do the unthinkable.

"I want you to go to her autopsy," he said.

He was a gentle and wise Jewish physician from Poland who had escaped the horrors of the Holocaust and who was instrumental in the development of American cardiology in the 50s and 60s. He relied on data and facts like any physician, but he also always listened to stories with the ear of a natural storyteller. He knew how close I had become to this family, but his inquisitive and brilliant mind also knew that her disease had something to teach me—something beyond the science of the disease.

"I can't do that," I said. "Please let someone else go in there to examine her heart and get the information we need." I thought, "Take this cup from me."

But he wouldn't. Despite the fact that I was an emotional wreck, he insisted.

And so I went. I went and held her still heart in my hands, the same one that I had cherished in life when it was filled with warm blood and beating with vigor.

I felt like a traitor.

But, gradually, that feeling changed. In its place was a growing sense of warmth and respect and love—the same feelings that I'd had for her in life. In that moment, she and I became connected once again beyond death.

I realized that her gift to me wasn't limited by what I had learned from her and her family in her lifetime. Her gift was timeless, boundless. I knew there was no turning back for me. I finally began to see how I might survive in the world of medicine and loss. And it caused me to rethink what I knew about medicine.

Should we allow ourselves the risk of loving and caring for patients?

My generation of physicians was taught to steel ourselves to loss, to withhold our emotions and our grief, to maintain our clinical, detached demeanor. We learned to shrug our shoulders, turn our faces away from terror and fear, and put on our white coats like amulets to protect us from the pain of our patients. We throw in the emotional towel and long for release from the agony that this work often entails. But I think this was the worst model we could have ever learned. None of this works.

I realized that the detachment from patients that I'd been taught to seek is a shallow approach. In fact, shutting down—sterilizing myself emotionally so that I don't feel anything— is far more painful than death itself. It turns patients into numbers and charts, and it empties lives of meaning. It renders patients dead and lifeless before their time. The nuances of the human heart cannot be captured in the sterility of medical records nor by simple intellectual preparations.

A well-known Jewish philosopher, Martin Buber, talked about this distinction between what he called an "I-It" relationship and an "I-Thou" relationship.[9] An "I-It" relationship is developed simply for a transactional benefit; we treat the other person as an "it." I fear this describes many patient/physician relationships; often physicians see patients as one of many transactions they face every day, in addition to insurance companies, employees, health systems, and the government. But when we behave as if the patient is simply an "it," we lose something of the inherent holiness of the healing vocation.

An "I-Thou" relationship, on the other hand, is what Buber considered one of the cornerstones of life.

---

9   Martin Buber, *I and Thou*, (New York: Scribner, 1978).

It is a meaningful relationship, a living, holy, honest entity. Perhaps—just perhaps—if we regain this sense of the "thou" of patient care, we can all leave our days in medicine with a higher sense of purpose and fulfillment than many are experiencing now.

I also understood for the very first time that, while I'm committed to sound science and wonderful technology, I also have to listen to stories. I have to learn what patients often have to teach us; I have to weave their stories into my own life.

And I learned that it's fine to be sad and to weep. Sure it hurts. So what? It is perfectly acceptable to become wounded and to mourn in medicine. There is a time to grieve. There is also a time to let go, to take what we have been given and learn, and to move forward with memories in love.

It's survivable. More importantly, it's worth it.

THE MOST POWERFUL
WORDS IN MEDICINE

What does it mean when prayers for healing seem to be met with profound silence?

Years ago, I heard an Anglican priest and renowned nuclear scientist named Reverend John Polkinghorne speak. A leading voice in the movement to reconcile science and religion, Rev. Polkinghorne recounted the tale of a close colleague at Cambridge who was diagnosed with pancreatic cancer. His friend had learned that he had no more than six months to live, and so he asked friends and colleagues to pray for his healing. They did. They gathered faithfully every morning and prayed for him. They prayed and prayed and *prayed*.

Six months later, he died.

At his funeral, his wife called Rev. Polkinghorne aside. She told him what may be the most powerful words in medicine.

"I want you to know," she said firmly, "that my husband died healed."

These are powerful words. Perhaps the *most* powerful in medicine. They matter because they fly in the face of what a lot of us are privately thinking. When our prayers are not answered and someone dies, we assume there is something wrong.

We may assume that it's because we are sinners—that we aren't good enough to be healed. Perhaps the illness, we reason, is a punishment from God. Every so often, someone will voice these private assumptions out loud, so I have quite a collection of these sayings from over the years.

But I call all of these sayings "BBT," or Bad Bedside Theology. They often reflect a past perceived experience with a harsh, judgmental, angry God. They all attempt to put the God of mystery into a small, vengeful box at the bedside in the presence of tragedy. Unfortunately, they have caused enormous damage on countless people of good will and faith. These sayings are all a misunderstanding of the nature of healing and the power of prayer.

The patient's wife in Rev. Polkinghorne's story intuitively knew the truth about prayer and healing. In spite of the evidence—after six months of seemingly unanswered prayers and at her husband's funeral no less—she was *assured* that her husband was healed. So what is it she knew?

What does it mean when prayers for healing seem to be met with profound silence?

For starters, the patient's wife understood that *healing* and *curing* are not the same. People mistakenly use these terms interchangeably, resulting in a morass of misunderstanding and pain for numerous patients.

Curing is about biology. But *healing* is about something fundamentally different.

To understand the difference, let's take a look at the origins of the words "to heal." One is *haelen*, an Old English word. It means "to bring fragments back to wholeness, to restore." Another origin comes from the Latin word *salvus,* which is the root for "salvation." So healing has nothing to do with a cure. It has everything to do with our journey to completion, our home in the fullness of creation.

This understanding has important implications for us as physicians.

When patients mistake healing for curing and begin spouting "BBT," wise clinicians will not necessarily want to counter these claims in the heat of the moment. They can act as "counterweights," allowing grieving families to experience something more loving, open, and forgiving at the bedside. Physicians cannot, of course, change a lifetime of religious perspectives but *can* gently move families into a healthier, more realistic place where suffering and grief is honored and respected.

We can also check our expectations for prayer. Many people pray to God as some sort of cosmic Santa Claus. Without even realizing it, they measure the effectiveness of prayer like some sort of celestial batting average. If they bat, say, more than .330, they have a good prayer season.

But it's not about winning or losing a "batting season." It's not about the number of prayer requests that are granted for cures. It is about transformation from brokenness to wholeness. It is about the mystery of healing and the power of moving into a relationship with the divine. It is *always* about healing and rarely about curing.

Our prayer life is liberated when we understand this crucial difference. Our expectations of our healthcare system are liberated as well. When we understand the truth about healing, we are freed to engage the journey of suffering in a new way. Even in the midst of the dark valley of the shadow of death, we can say yes to life. Suffering, then, becomes not something that defines us or limits us—it becomes a crucible that heals us and moves us back into relationship with God and those closest to us.

And this is what the widow of Polkinghorne's colleague knew. The biology of the disease took its inevitable course, as it often does. Her husband was not cured, and yet it did not have the final say. The parts of his life that were broken, wounded, or incomplete had been made whole again. In his journey toward death, he made peace with colleagues and family.

He was healed.

LET GO

What can we learn from our belief systems during times of trial?

In 1972, I spent the summer working as a medical volunteer in Honduras for an international healthcare organization called Amigos de Las Americas. Our group went from village to village in the mountains near El Salvador, often seeing up to 200 patients a day. These patients would walk for hours or even days to see the physician, so I didn't have the heart to tell them that I was only a senior in medical school.

Toward the end of my third week there, we visited a tiny village where a parade was in progress. People marched through the dirt streets, singing songs and playing music. They held hands and lifted their eyes heavenward.

At the end of the procession, a tiny coffin was carried aloft on the shoulders of village men. As I watched with curiosity, I found out that the coffin held the body of a four-year-old child. She had died just the day before after getting a minor cut.

I stared in shock. "We could have saved her," I found myself muttering in sadness and frustration. Our group possessed all the supplies and medication that easily could have treated her infection, but we were just forty-eight hours too late. "We could have saved her life. Children shouldn't die from simple lacerations!"

I was devastated.

"All of our work is in vain!" I thought in despair. "Why do we even bother if this is to be the fate of the people after we leave?"

As I raged at the injustice, I watched the family and friends of the little girl. These people dealt with tragedy daily, and they carried themselves with a quiet dignity. They were grieving, yet they were also celebrating life— and each other. All around me, I saw only love.

In that moment, I realized this is where faith comes in. I'm not talking about the faith of Sunday school lessons, catechisms, or televangelists. I'm talking about faith that is real, lived, and visceral—the kind that survives the tragedies that would bring many Americans to an angry, wounded despair.

What can we learn from our belief systems during times of trial?

When grappling with pain and suffering, the early Greek Christian fathers used the word, *apathei*. It is often totally misunderstood in modern times because it's mistakenly translated as "apathy," which means indifference or lack of caring. But the true meaning of *apathei* is nothing of the sort.

Apathei is a wise and healthy "letting go." It is a letting go of pain and suffering and the need to control outcomes. It is an expression of total trust of the divine presence in our lives, an act of simply letting God be God. As Jesus said in Luke 9:60, "Let the dead bury the dead." *Apathei* is acknowledging that we are ultimately not in charge, a simple fact that may be the hardest for many of us to grasp.

But as healthcare professionals exposed to immense suffering and seemingly random pain, we must grasp the truth about *apathei*. We are called to confront suffering, but then we must let it go. We have to let suffering become a comma in our vocation, not a period. When we wisely close the emotional door on our wounds and pick up the pieces of our questions, we are able to return to work. It is the only way to find the strength to remain faithful to the gifts that we are given daily in the world of medicine.

In this profession, we *will* come across tragedies that sweep us away and leave us adrift emotionally. But an understanding of *apathei* helps us to step out of our despair to see the bigger picture, which is this: life and death are always together in this world, and it is our privilege to simply be witness to it all. We are a part of everything it means to be human, including suffering. We cannot expect or demand to avoid suffering. Both human brokenness *and* grace flow equally into our lives as physicians. A Buddhist anecdote, known as a Zen koan, might embrace the notion that one has to both attach *and* detach to be fully human.

This truth was made clear to me just two weeks

after the death of the little girl. We had been traveling all day in a four-wheel drive vehicle until there was no more mud trail to follow. Then we got out, loaded our supplies on the backs of mules, and marched single-file up into the mountains. At dusk in the valley below, we glimpsed a tiny village of a few huts and a simple chapel. I hadn't eaten all day and was famished, fatigued, and still running on emotional fumes.

As we descended into the village, we found a woman waiting for us. She motioned for me to follow her to the end of a path, where there was a tiny hut surrounded by women holding candles. A teenage girl was inside. She had been in labor for more than twenty-four hours and had sky-high blood pressure. Her temperature was 103 degrees. Even with the best that modern medicine had to offer, I knew that this girl and her child were likely to die. But I'd had enough of death.

Without electricity, running water, or lights of any kind, and with nothing but a dirt floor, I got to work. I started an intravenous line and performed a small surgical procedure to facilitate the delivery. And then, an hour later, life asserted itself in the unlikeliest of places. A beautiful, healthy boy burst into the world. And with him, overcoming my despair, burst an unexpected moment of grace.

It is an unexpected moment of grace like this that is a gift for physicians. It is a healing balm that allows us to survive other devastating encounters. We rely on moments like this to pull us above our darkest despair and sustain us with hope, joy, and faith.

WAY OFF SCRIPT

Can medical training fully prepare physicians for tragic situations?

It began as a normal Sunday, typically a quiet day at Hillcrest Baptist Medical Center and Providence Hospital in Waco, Texas. But the events that unfolded that day would irrevocably change my life, the lives of all my colleagues, and those of our entire community.

It was February 28, 1993, a day marking the beginning of the siege on the Mount Carmel Center, which was a mere nine miles north of Waco. The U.S. Bureau of Alcohol, Tobacco and Firearms (ATF) raided the center as part of an investigation into illegal possession of firearms and explosives. A two-hour gun battle ensued between the ATF and a religious sect called Branch Davidians, led by David Koresh, a man who believed himself to be the final prophet. The firefight resulted in the deaths of four agents and six Branch Davidians, and the FBI Hostage Rescue Team would attempt to negotiate with Koresh over the next fifty-one days.

From the time of the initial assault on the compound, emergency rooms throughout the region were thrown into chaos. Most of our staff had no direct knowledge of what was transpiring at Mount Carmel Center, yet we suddenly found ourselves at the center of national attention. Lawyers were already a palpable presence; the media was everywhere they could get without a pass.

Before we had time to collect ourselves, we were facing the wounded, dying, and dead. The hospital corridors suddenly looked like war zones. Each patient was assigned an armed guard. There were bloody bandages on innocent victims and on federal agents alike. Some patients screamed with pain from near-fatal burns. The physicians, many with no training in combat medicine, were triaging the wounded and fatalities. The families were stunned into silence, their hollow, vacant eyes filled with fear.

It was all very surreal. My medical training equipped me for data collection and problem-solving, but this?

Can medical training fully prepare physicians for tragic situations?

As I took in the devastation around me, I realized we were way off script. Even the best medical education in the world could not have prepared me for this.

My education hadn't prepared me to hear the intimate details of life inside the compound by one of the victims. She was a woman in her mid-fifties, a gentle and kind soul who was released by Koresh and suffering from severe congestive heart failure. She was not a member of the cult but a visitor from Guyana on an extended study period, quite literally "caught in the crossfire" of the siege. She recounted to me stories of sexual abuse of minors, mixed in paradoxically enough with seemingly innocent Biblical wisdom. Their brand of "wisdom" was a strange blend of violence and apocalyptic ideology, held by people who wanted to live apart from a world that they believed was decaying.

Medical education also hadn't prepared me for the other areas of involvement that were asked of me. After we stabilized her heart, the woman asked me to be her conduit to the US District Attorney. I worked with the two of them to fill in some of the missing elements of the drama that remained a work in progress. This was not covered in Patient/Physician Relationships 101!

My training hadn't prepared me for the lengths some journalists will go to in order to get inside information. I was "passing the peace" at church when I turned to a man with a friendly smile, clearly a visitor, who said, "The peace of the Lord be with you." He also handed me his business card and asked me to appear on his nationally syndicated morning show the next morning. I have nothing but the highest regard for members of any branch of journalism, for they are truly the conduit for the most pressing issues of our times, but this experience left me a bit dismayed.

Even the press conferences that are often necessary in these situations left me feeling woefully unprepared. Each day, I gave a daily progress report on my patients' conditions, but I found it hard to be factual while not divulging details about our patients and breaching confidentiality. It was especially hard to remain calm and objective on camera in the midst of immense suffering, injustice, and loss.

The siege came to a tragic end on April 19, 1993, when the building caught on fire. Seventy-nine Branch Davidians died that day, including twenty-two children.

The devastation that Koresh unleashed may have been stopped, but in the aftermath of the siege, another insidious and silent tragedy began to unfold. The physicians and nurses who had cared for the victims and witnessed the devastation began to struggle. Confronting the violence and death took an inevitable toll on everyone's souls and psyches. I realized that we were all entering new territory, one in which the victims are not only the patients but the healthcare teams themselves.

The issues that arise for caregivers who are on duty in times of tragedy are well documented. They can manifest as anything from mild generalized anxiety to full-blown post-traumatic stress disorder. These can lead to a paralysis of the spirit and a questioning of one's future in the world of health care. And these issues can last. To this day, many of my nursing colleagues—those who were working in the ER with the wounded and dead victims—remain scarred by the memories of loss and senseless death. That event defined our lives in ways that are still hard to describe.

I learned in a very real and vivid way that life rarely follows a script, and, therefore, neither does medicine. Medical education is often mechanized and routine, but it doesn't touch reality. The reality is that medicine does not exist in a vacuum; it often stands at the crossroads of culture, mirroring our national soul and conscience. It is part of the very woof and warp of the lives around us, including the lives that were there that day of the siege in Waco as well as the lives today who are impacted by mass school shootings.

I also learned this: no matter how strong, resilient, and centered we physicians think we are, we have our limits. And when we do meet our limits, we encounter what many writers have called the "dark night of the soul." This is where physicians and other healthcare providers are forced to look into the shadows of human existence. It's not a pretty thing. It can lead one into the vortex of doubt, anger, resentment, and recrimination. The dark night of the soul is where we doubt our calling, where we experience pain beyond that which we think we can endure. It's where we ask questions to which there are no answers. And it's where we share the burden of what it means to suffer in the midst of unexplained violence.

Of course, these are normal and healthy feelings. They are affirmed in many blog sites and books by healthcare professionals and other caregivers, including a wonderful book titled, *Pain Seeking Understanding: Suffering, Medicine, and Faith*.[10] In it, Deborah Healey, a pediatrician who has encountered cases of unimaginable abuse, describes her own dark night of the soul. She

---

10   Margaret Mohrmann, *Pain Seeking Understanding: Suffering, Medicine, and Faith*, (Ohio: Pilgrim Press, 1999).

says, "There have been times in my life when it was hard to hear more stories of suffering, to carry more burdens. My own woes competed for my attention and even threatened to overwhelm me. I found God absent, not there to buoy me up. At those times, I could not do my work."

"At the same time," she goes on, "I cannot avoid coming up against evil. I can shun it, but it is nevertheless all around us at every level of existence. I must choose to acknowledge the evil and confront it directly if I am going to provide the care sought of me as a doctor to share the suffering and to ease the burdens of my patients."

I have found that, paradoxically, it is by embracing the loss of others that we find a common ground of humanity that is almost holy. It connects us to our patients in ways that are beyond imagination. In fact, these shared moments of grace in the midst of loss are what kept me afloat in my own dark night of the soul, in the days and hours when I didn't have the strength to do this any longer. I have found that these purest, most real, most authentic encounters often occur in the losses, not in the victories, providing a firm foundation for healers in times of transitions in our system.

For Healey, her faith is what has helped her endure these times and continue to function. She says, "I could not bear the burdens alone. I had to find healing for myself, to reconnect with God before I could presume once again to offer care to others. . . . I can do this day after day only with God's help, by being open to knowing God's will from my patients and through my connections to them, and open to receiving the precious moments of grace."

As physicians, we are not fully prepared for tragic situations. When facing horror, we are likely to lose our wonderful but naïve optimism. We may even lose ourselves for a time in a dark night of the soul. In these crises, may we acknowledge our limits and allow our own wounds to heal. May we seek pastoral counseling, which provides a firm foundation in the wake of spiritual stress, and which I can attest has saved more than one career in medicine. And may we rely on our faith to continue to provide a light for our patients in a dark world.

RESURRECTION

How does death give life?

The patient lying before me was a wonderful college senior who had fainted in the shower one day before graduation. By all outward appearances, she'd had a simple fainting spell, the kind that thousands of people have every day due to nothing more than stress.

But it wasn't that simple. When this young woman wore a portable heart monitor, we detected life-threatening rhythm problems. We knew she was at risk for SCD, or sudden cardiac death syndrome. In the past, SCD was a death sentence. There was no pharmaceutical solution for this condition that caused the deaths of many young athletes during competition. And there was no way to project which patients could die and which would simply faint then regain consciousness.

But now, with the marvels of engineering, technology, and research, we're provided a whole new field of devices that literally save lives, including the defibrillator we were implanting in the chest of this young woman. It is capable of allowing young and old alike to live far beyond tragically foreshortened life expectancies.

The defibrillator charged in a few seconds. It was storing enough energy in a capacitor to deliver a small shock to the patient's heart.

In some ways, this technology makes perfect sense. Devices like this defibrillator merely take advantage of predictable properties of physics and biology to help us help our patients. All molecules born in the primordial chaos of the Big Bang have, over time, emerged as the wonder of the human condition. In a very literal way, we are made up of matter that is recycled and rearranged.

But it goes beyond that. We're *more* than simply matter that is recycled and rearranged. People of faith acknowledge that we are imprinted with *imago dei*, Latin for "the image of God," which we call our soul. We're matter that has been *transformed* by something very spiritual into this miracle of humanity. It is because of this transformation that many spiritual traditions call for dying to oneself in order to experience life again. While dying to oneself may not end in heroics or survival as we tend to define it, it opens the door to a rebirth of sorts that outlives our biological existence.

That's what makes this technology so profound. Much of our biomedical research consists of harnessing the properties and energy of a universe that is "wonderfully and fearfully made," including the process of recycling, rearrangement, and transformation.[11] The best research always draws upon these deep insights

---

11   *New American Standard Bible* © 1995, Psalm 139:14.

into the human condition and follows a journey to healing where technology is used with wisdom and compassion.

Therefore, much of medicine is about life emerging from the darkness of a tomb. It's about being born again. It is about willingly dying to oneself in order to be resurrected. Of course, this power and gift can be both misused and misinterpreted by families and providers alike. But more often than not, we do a good thing when we bring life from death.

How does death give life?

This concept is part of the predictable, profound order of the universe. In order to save our patients, to make them live, we sometimes have to make them die first. This is why we take a scalpel to cut away good tissue. It's why we give patients chemotherapy. Quite literally, we are trying to kill them in order to save their lives.

We're counting on the fact that cutting away good tissue allows us to remove cancerous tissue. We're betting that killing diseased bone marrow will give birth to healthy cells. Over and over, we are called to die in the world of medicine, only to be reborn again.

This is why we were using a defibrillator with this young woman. We were hoping that stopping her heart would allow it to beat again. We completed the implant, turned on the power, and allowed a surge of electricity into her body.

A few tense seconds passed, and then . . . her heart monitor produced a blessed "beep."

It worked. Her heart had restarted. I exhaled and waited for my own heart to stop racing.

This was a small, daily miracle of modern technology, yet it didn't fail to make my spirit give thanks. I had always viewed medicine as a place where one's theology meets the road, and now I knew it to be true.

From death, life emerged stronger than ever. A young woman was reborn.

EVERYDAY
SACRAMENTS

How do we find meaning in the ordinary?

It's 2 a.m. in the Intensive Care Unit, and everything is still and quiet. Voices are hushed.

Families from out of town are camped in the waiting room, making it look different. It's like a cross between a campground and a battlefield.

At this hour, even the sounds of the hospital itself seem different. The most compelling is the quiet, steady rise and fall of the respirator. Unlike the older, louder generations of respirators, this newer model emits sounds that are so very gentle, almost peaceful. It seems to puff effortlessly, very much like my own breath. *Inhale, exhale. Inhale, exhale.*

It's all very ordinary, and yet . . . these small sights and sounds move me.

How do we find meaning in the ordinary?

It starts with our perspective. Take, for instance, that waiting room and this respirator that are such ordinary parts of hospital life. To me, they are anything but ordinary. They are glimpses of the divine.

You see, families are often reunited in waiting rooms such as this one. Amid the clutter of lumpy sleeping bags and personal belongings, loved ones bond with each other as they desperately cling to hope. And this respirator—it's pumping the most basic necessity of life. This great gift of technology is moving oxygen in and out of a human body, literally giving the breath of life.

Some might laugh at the suggestion that these things are divine, chalking it up to sleep deprivation. Others may be offended. Only the celestial music of J.S. Bach, they might say, is the true expression of the divine.

But we make a huge ontological mistake when we think that only glorious art or music can be a gateway to the mystery of the holy. It can be a very simple, seemingly mundane sound. A respirator, perhaps, or a baby's crying breath. It's a moment that unexpectedly wakes up our soul at some primal level.

The Hebrew word for this glimpse of the divine is *ruah,* which translates as "spirit wind," or "breath of God." The New Testament Greek, in its attempt to capture the mystery of the divine nature, often pairs the word *pneuma,* or "vital spirit," with the descriptive term "holy." Over the ages, we have understood that this holy, energizing life force sustains us in times of life and death, in times of hope and despair. The sound of the respirator is simply the sound of the Spirit entering into the heart of the healthcare encounter with incredible power.

We are given these divine glimpses and, in many ways, they are pure sacraments. I'm not talking about the official sacraments that are recognized by Christians, like baptism and communion, which are the two constant examples through the millennia. I'm talking about sacraments as they are described in the working definition, "an outward and visible sign of an inward and spiritual grace." In this way, to me, these divine glimpses are as sacramental as baptism and communion.

This is what I was thinking the first time I witnessed an organ transplant. I'd thought I was sure of what to expect, but I was brought my knees in awe of something holy and amazing.

The operating theater combined a sense of purposeful activity and profound respect. There was a low hum of muted voices, and some gentle classical music was playing in the background.

Members from the local operating room team worked in conjunction with a group that had flown in to receive the harvested organs.

Incisions were made swiftly. For a change, the anesthesiologist was not concerned with sedation so much as stabilizing the vital signs so the organs maintained adequate perfusion during the procedure, essentially keeping the organs alive.

Carefully, one by one, important organs were removed and prepared to continue their journey into the life of another human being. Heart, lungs, liver, kidneys, bones, corneas, skin . . . all were used in some capacity. It all was handled gently and tenderly with deep respect for the person whose earthly journey was ending.

At the end of the procedure, machines were turned off. One life ended. Another was getting a second chance.

All of us in that room sensed that we were a part of an infinite, divine journey. A sacrament. I think everyone there regardless of their religious views knew that their skills were a part of something truly eternal. The whole process had been efficient, gentle, dedicated, and breathtaking. It embodied the best that medicine can offer, and it made me deeply grateful to be a part of the tradition of healing. A few moments of silence were shared, and then, one at a time, the physicians, nurses, and technicians moved on to the next part of their daily responsibilities.

Years later, when my sister-in-law was to receive a heart-double-lung transplant, I thought back to the awe and mystery of that sacramental moment in the operating theater. My sister-in-law was preparing for a miracle that we now take for granted, one that allowed her an additional decade of life she needed to raise a young son. Still today, I continue to be surprised by glimpses of the divine. These moments don't always have the official sanction of the church; indeed, more often than not, they are found in the most ordinary, daily encounters.

This point is made beautifully by author and theologian Leonardo Boff in his book, *Sacraments of Life:*

Life of Sacraments.[12] His captivating book cover portrays a loaf of bread, a cigarette butt, and a cup of coffee. Inside, Boff explains that anything that brings us into the presence of God has the power to become a sacrament, including the three seemingly simple objects on his book cover. For him, the bread, cigarette, and coffee bring him into the presence of his dead father, who had introduced him to his faith in South America. From these objects, it is a short leap for Boff to the presence of something holy: the divine Spirit living and breathing in the midst of human brokenness and suffering.

Sacraments aren't always objects like the three on Boff's cover. Even people *themselves* become living sacraments: the sound of voices communicating love, the touch of family members or physicians and nurses. These sacraments remind us that God can be found in this created, rather earthy, messy world where people live, breathe, and work. They provide the gift of vision, of seeing the world in a new and life-affirming way.

Whether they are objects or people, I have been reminded again and again throughout my medical career about the power of sacraments in our everyday lives. And over a lifetime in medicine, I have found it is often the "small" things that move me the most. The big dramatic scenes are certainly memorable, but they do not make up the lion's share of a physician's working life. It is in the daily rhythms, ebbs, and flows of a hospital that I find my work to be the most intriguing and ultimately satisfying.

---

12   Leonardo Boff, *Sacraments of Life: Life of Sacraments*, (Oregon: Pastoral Press, 1998).

As healthcare professionals, we must recognize and acknowledge sacraments wherever and whenever we find them. They *are* there, waiting for us to notice. And they are never more plainly recognizable than in the cluttered mess of a waiting room . . . in the elegance of an organ transplantation . . . and in the mundane, miraculous rise and fall of a respirator.

THE
PATIENT

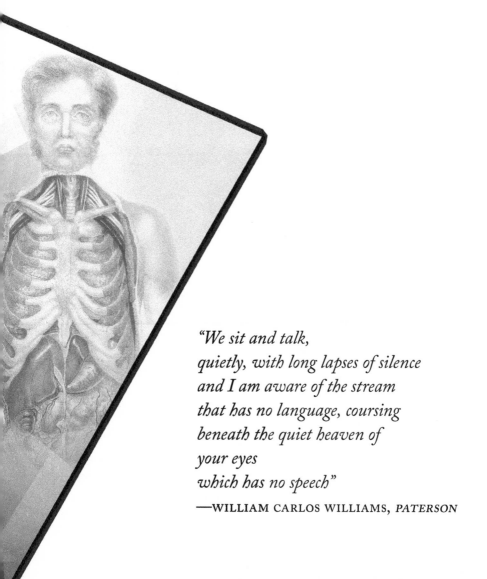

"We sit and talk,
quietly, with long lapses of silence
and I am aware of the stream
that has no language, coursing
beneath the quiet heaven of
your eyes
which has no speech"

—WILLIAM CARLOS WILLIAMS, *PATERSON*

BROKEN IN BODY
AND SPIRIT

How can patients break the downward cycle of grief?

It is a leaching out of the marrow of our lives. At times it starts with a bang or a catastrophic and unpredictable event. At other times it dribbles away drop by drop into an ocean of tears. I'm talking about grieving the loss of a loved one. And in either case—whether it is sudden or prolonged—the loss of a loved one brings patients to the heart of their own darkness and despair.

Whether the loss is due to a disease, accident, or self-inflicted end, it leads to pain that most people cannot get their heads and hearts around. And in the aftermath, they are left to somehow survive these tragedies that defy description. Words of comfort often fail, and desolation seems to rip apart everything that they know to be true about life, death, and God.

As they pick up the rubble of their lives, people have their ways of responding to existential pain and suffering. Elizabeth Kubler-Ross outlined the five stages of grief that people generally follow: denial, anger, bargaining, depression, and acceptance.[13] And, as a physician, I would agree that there is great value in understanding these five stages as a normal journey that is a part of all humanity.

But these five stages also seem to minimize grief. That's because true grief wrecks more than emotions. The reality is that our bodies translate emotional pain and loss into *physical* pain. I have heard patients describe real physical symptoms during major periods of grief.

I am reminded of a woman I treated many years ago who experienced those symptoms. She had lost her husband three years previously, and yet her grief persisted. She was perched at the end of the bed, shoulders slumped. There was a whiteness to her knuckles, and her palms glistened. One eye twitched as we talked.

"My chest is really hurting. You have no idea how bad I'm feeling," she said, a tear emerging from one eye and dropping quietly." She brushed it away impatiently. "I know this is just a part of grieving that I'm going through. I'll be fine soon."

But I knew she would not be fine soon. Her grief was manifesting itself physically. Her body was loaded with signals that all pointed to an impending physical crisis triggered by loss.

I think many initial clinical visits are a result of people thinking like this woman. They do not understand their bodies nor how they respond to stress. They do not know that their bodies are wired to respond in a certain way that is common. They often experience chest constriction,

---

13   Elizabeth Kubler-Ross, *On Death and Dying*, (New York: Scribner, 1997).

dizziness, sweating, nausea, palpitations, neck and back pains, headaches, and weakness. Often their physical symptoms persist for longer than they would like, which is what ultimately leads some patients to seek medical attention. Unfortunately, it is all too easy for physicians to commonly dismiss these symptoms as psychosomatic.

But I firmly believe that grief is not only in our heads but also in our bodies. This is borne out by research in the area of grief and its biologic effects. New brain imaging technology and biochemical analysis demonstrate that grief and loss trigger the release of pro-inflammatory cytokines and alter our biological defense mechanisms. These are the very same substances that are now linked to heart attacks, strokes, and other illnesses. They may actually affect the immune system in a negative way, allowing cells to mutate and divide, setting the stage for serious cardiac disease or cancer.

Not only that, but grieving individuals behave much like people exposed to the addictive effects of cocaine. Neurological receptors are activated and, after the first exposure, addiction is a certainty. Loss may trigger the same downward cycle of physiological responses that lead to protracted grief *and* the possibility of new disease.

How can patients break the spiral of grief?

First, we should understand that grief extends beyond the five emotional stages. There is an immunologi-cal component to grief. When our bodies experience strange sensations after devastating loss, it should be seen as much more profound than the experience of psychological trauma. It is our bodies' way of sending warning signals to the brain that something radical is going on in our bodies. It is a wake-up call.

Second, we—patients and physicians alike—must honor and not deny these very real physical symptoms of our grief. This acceptance allows us to take steps toward healing. An approach such as this subtly bucks the compartmentalization that is used in science, religion, and sometimes even by our families. Science and religion try to break us down into components that make sense, and our families welcome the tidy confines of understanding. But we must respect our grief and not suppress it. This includes learning to decipher our body signals with wisdom, compassion, and grace. Failure to do so means that we only compound the problem.

Third, we need to be aware that it is not only mourning that can trigger these things. Any devastating loss can trigger the same neurochemical and anatomical responses. It can be the loss of a meaningful relationship with a dear friend, a divorce, the loss of a job, a relocation because of a job transfer—even an illness. In a tangible way, an illness challenges us to grieve the loss of our health, vigor, and youth. Disease robs us of something we value. We move from the "Kingdom of Health" into the "Kingdom of Illness," and our lives are forever altered.

Finally, we must *face* the darkness—and this is perhaps the hardest of all. We have to embrace the sorrow and loss that is within us. We must acknowledge our body signals and express words of grief, rage, terror, helplessness, or blind frustration. It all comes with the territory. We cannot hide from sorrow.

In the end, when faced with the horror of grief, we also come face to face with our own finitude. We must accept that, in that place of profound loss, we are broken in both body *and* spirit. Yes, we may find our way back to familiar routines and patterns, but we should hold dearly to the understanding that something very deep about our lives will never be the same. And as we honor our grief as part of the fabric of our lives, may we eventually find our way back to lives of meaning.

ROAD RAGE OF
THE BODY

What are the effects of forgiveness on health care?

There is a human tendency that can unleash a plethora of diseases and physiological disasters. It's often the major component of heart attacks, ulcers, strokes, and neuromuscular problems—and these outcomes are just the tip of the iceberg. This condition is a veritable road rage of the body, making health care difficult for physicians to facilitate until it is addressed.

The condition is unforgiveness. Clinical practitioners have seen firsthand the devastating effects of repressed anger, hostility, and an unwillingness to forgive.

And the anecdote? It's not sophisticated treatments and medicines. The anecdote is forgiveness.

In an article titled, "Forgiveness in Health Research and Medical Practice," in *Explore: The Journal of Science and Healing*, the authors say, "Forgiveness is an ancient concept. It is a mark of compassion, love and caring, and is enshrined in all the great religions as a gesture of supreme value . . . and is a natural concern for the healing professions."[14] Indeed, over the last decade, there has been a growing body of research on the intimate connection between what we think, feel, and believe and how our bodies respond to illness, disease, or stress.

The notion of forgiveness as strictly a theological concern is now moving into the practical world of clinical medicine and bedside patient care. There is increasing evidence suggesting forgiveness may be one of the underlying paradigms that promote biological and physiological change and, ultimately, healing. There is so much evidence, in fact, that research on forgiveness is now part of mainstream medicine. Harvard Medical School, Scripps Research Institute, and others are funding the development of fulltime programs of research into the mind-body connection. From the research, it seems that three practical implications of forgiveness have emerged.

What are the effects of forgiveness on health care?

Physicians need to know that one effect of forgiveness is its role in reducing medical malpractice litigation. Studies have confirmed that medical malpractice suits are not usually triggered by bad outcomes or medical mistakes. Their real origin is wherever there is distrust and a lack of communication. A major study

---

14   Everett Worthington, et al. "Forgiveness in Health Research and Medical Practice." *Explore: The Journal of Science and Healing*, no. 3 (May 2005): 169-176, https://doi.org/10.1016/j.explore.2005.02.012.

recently showed that one of the strongest, most proactive acts a physician can do when a mistake is made is to honestly address it with patients and families, asking their forgiveness when appropriate. The risk of litigation seems to be reduced by the human act of forgiveness, which is a quantum shift from the past when mistakes were not addressed frankly.

Beyond malpractice issues, patients need to truly let go of wounds, real or perceived, that are caused by others. This seems to produce measurable anatomical and physiological benefits. Brain scans done before and after simple meditative forgiveness exercises show remarkable beneficial effects on brain function, white blood cell action, inflammation, and immunological responsiveness. Our bodies seem to be hard-wired to forgive others. Evolutionary biologists postulate certain evolutionary advantages because holding on to anger clearly has a negative effect on individual and community survival curves.

Patients also need to forgive themselves. This is something all religious traditions teach and honor, and it's how they will find their true center where healing occurs. Alcoholics Anonymous calls it "making amends" for the transgressions they commit.[15] We all have places where we need to hold ourselves lightly—to be accountable but also to gently let go of the hurt we have caused others. Forgiving ourselves is difficult, but studies now

---

15   Alcoholics Anonymous World Services, *Twelve Steps and Twelve Traditions,* (New York: AA Worldwide Services, 2002), 83-87: https://www.aa.org/assets/en_US/en_step9.pdf.

affirm that unless we can let go of that guilt, we set our bodies up for unfortunate biomedical consequences.

Ultimately, forgiveness is foundational to the practice of medicine. Physicians can facilitate the process by foregoing expensive testing and simply being willing to listen and gently learn from what patients say is important in their lives. And patients can move toward health by first forgiving themselves and then forgiving others. This is where healing begins.

GOOD VIBRATIONS

How is music a catalyst for healing?

Thirty-five years ago, I was a resident with a man who became one of my closest friends. We did nearly everything together. We took care of dying patients together and shared our hopes and dreams in medicine. We prayed together and laughed together. We had our hearts broken more than once together. And when we got married, our wives went through pregnancies together. Our sons were even born only a few days apart.

But that is where our experiences diverged. My son came into the world in perfect health; my friend's son did not. His son was born with a deadly congenital heart condition. He survived multiple corrective surgeries and outlived his poor early prognosis, and then, while walking down the hall of his high school just a few weeks before graduation, he collapsed and died.

After his death, my friend and his wife channeled their grief in productive ways as part of their own journey to healing. He became the director of a large regional hospice program in Kentucky. She earned a master's degree in music therapy and specialized in music as a healing modality for terminally ill patients.

It was their personal experience and specialized knowledge that prompted me to invite my friend and his wife to present their story at a Medical Humanities retreat at Baylor University. When they arrived, she produced a small harp and told the group of pre-med students that it was the very harp she uses to play tunes for dying patients. She explained that she places the harp directly on the chest of each patient. When she plays, the patient feels the vibrations of the strings, and, even in the midst of death, their bodies respond to various frequencies and sensations. Invariably, deep peace and calm enter the realm of clinical medicine.

The combination of her skills as a musician and her husband's gifts as a clinician were bringing hope and peace to countless patients under their care. While virtually all of their patients are terminal, nearly all die in a state of healing.

How is music a catalyst for healing?

My friends were tapping into what Albert Einstein discovered: that matter and energy are part of the same unified reality. Every piece of matter in the universe vibrates or oscillates at a certain frequency. From humans to stars to seemingly inert matter, everything created at the instant of the Big Bang moves at its own particular pace and rhythm.

This phenomenon is at the forefront of our understanding of the world. For example, because crystals are tuned to their own frequency, we are able to use quartz as the fundamental substance around which to track time. It has a precise, predictable, and unfailing cycle length. And because different body parts vibrate at different frequencies, we can use magnetic resonance imaging (MRI) scanners to produce images of the human body in various states of health and disease. Molecular medicine and biology take advantage of this phenomenon to understand how humans are created and how we can facilitate their journey to healing.

Now, with a deeper understanding of the connection between vibration and healing, my students and I watched as my friend's wife placed her harp directly on each of our chests. We grew still, listening quietly as she played a few chords from J. S. Bach's "Be Thou My Vision." With the hum of each chord, we were transported to a different realm. We were connected to something beyond ourselves, to a place of transcendent peace and healing.

THE MYSTICAL POWER
OF PETS

How do animals heal us?

"I don't know how I could have gotten through this without Rosie," said my elderly patient.

I smiled, assuming she was referring to a dear friend, counselor, or pastor. As it turned out, "Rosie" was her dog.

As a clinician, I have observed that this isn't uncommon among elderly patients. I've learned that in many cases, it is an animal that provides them with companionship that may be missing in their lives. And in my medical practice, I occasionally witness the healing power of these relationships between patients and their animals.

How do animals heal us?

One way that animals play a role in healing is by impacting our memories of the past. Our memories are among the many things that define our human journey. We recall events, places, smells, textures, tastes, and loves lost and gained. In our religious lives, we institutionalize these memories, and they become rites that mark certain transformative events and that have the power to both honor our past and shape our future.

These memories often affect us in ways that are profound, yet unconscious. We know, for example, that repressed memories can hinder our journey to healing and wholeness. On the other hand, I've seen how positive memories help patients deal with disease, illness, tragedy, and death. Pets can play a part in reinforcing positive memories. They seem to evoke strong and deep memories, some surely personal and some even archetypical.

This impact of a pet on memories became evident when an elderly cat came to live with a friend of mine. The pet had belonged to a relative who had died of breast cancer. Although the cat could be a bit moody and aggressive from time to time—she was affectionately known as "psycho cat"—the animal served as a living bridge to the past. She reconnected them to memories of the family member they had lost. She was a living reminder of their storehouse of treasures. In time, my friend and his family forged memories of their own with the cat. Their pet became a part of the dynamic of healing for everyone—so much so that when the cat died, my friend grieved not only the loss of a part of the family but also a link to the past.

The mystical power of animals impacts more than the past; it can also influence our present. Animals give unconditional love and support when our own resources are depleted and need renewal. They divert our attention from our own needs to the needs of another. Perhaps most importantly, they help us continue to live in the moment.

But animals also shape our futures. I see this most clearly with service dogs who have been trained to interact with hospitalized patients. When these dogs arrive at the floor of the hospital, it is like witnessing a moment of concentrated love. Patients who haven't smiled or engaged in weeks are suddenly lit up from the inside. The mystical power of these animals stir an expectation of hope for the future, and these patients are often ready to take their first steps toward the journey of healing.

A LAUGHING MATTER

How does humor heal?

"Hearty laughter is a good way to jog internally without having to go outdoors," wrote Norman Cousins. He was a renowned political journalist, professor, and world peace advocate who published this profound statement in his pioneer work, *Anatomy of an Illness as Perceived by the Patient.*[16] It is about the power of humor, hope, and positive thinking on the ability of the body to heal in difficult circumstances. In it, he details how he learned from his own experience of disease and illness that laughter is intimately involved with the healing process.

When faced with a diagnosis of a potentially incapacitating and painful illness, Cousins' first response was to rent the collection of Marx Brothers films and watch them repeatedly. He soon found himself on the road to recovery and healing. He summarized the experience by writing, "I have learned to never underestimate the capacity of the human mind and body to regenerate."

---

16 Norman Cousins, *Anatomy of an Illness as Perceived by the Patient: Reflections on Healing and Regeneration,* (New York: Bantam Books, 1981).

Today, in a newer era of mind-body consciousness, we realize that Cousins' work was at the forefront of an understanding of the role of laughter in healing. Humor acknowledges our human frailties and allows us to laugh at ourselves, at the world, and at our suffering. It can function as an emotional safety valve in times of stress and illness.

Humor is as complex as the issues it regulates. Sometimes humor is mixed up in strange and wonderful ways with pathos and tragedy. The ancient Greek playwrights knew that. Actors would change their masks from smiley faces to sad faces, often in the same scene. Other times, humor borders on political incorrectness.

But I think that approaching these humorous and all-too-human moments with the judgment of a prim and proper Victorian perspective robs us of the healing power of laughter. Certainly we need to be respectful of others and their stories. But to try to sterilize the human condition is to deny it joy and magic. We must allow room for humor to heal, even when it points to that which we would rather not see.

How does humor heal?

For clinicians and healthcare providers, humor is like a dose of medicine. It allows them to laugh honestly at themselves and at the unbelievably funny things that they experience daily. Physicians who are willing to take themselves less seriously find themselves in a better place to reach out and enter the heart of pain, suffering, and laughter with their patients.

This comic relief explains the popularity of a book during my residency called *House of God*, written by a Harvard Medical School faculty member under a pen name, Dr. Samuel Shem.[17] It became the iconic symbol of the dark, humorous side of medical education and training. It vividly portrayed the workweek of 120-plus hours during which doctors are reduced to zombies and patients are seen as caricatures. It was funny, savage, sassy, and painfully difficult to read. It made fun of patients, medical students, interns, faculty, and the system itself. One medical school made it mandatory reading yet warned students not to read it until they graduated, for fear it could drive them away from medicine.

House of God was the literary precursor to such television shows as "Grey's Anatomy" and "House." In a strange and almost morbid way, it enabled many of us to simply survive the dehumanizing side of our education. It became an outlet for our sadness, tears, fears, and the raw side of our fragile egos and unmanageable lives.

Humor heals patients, as Norman Cousins discovered. In recent studies, we have discovered that humor activates positive aspects of our immune systems. This leads to better outcomes in terms of healing, even in risky medical procedures. I have seen patients who are willing to laugh at themselves recover better than those

---

17   Samuel Shem, House of God, (Pennsylvania: Richard Marek Publishers, 1978).

who face their circumstances with humorless stoicism. Some of the most poignant, funny, and beautiful stories I hear are from patients as they share their life experiences with full honesty. We share a laugh, and the healing begins—for the patient *and* for this physician.

MORE THAN
A PASTIME

What is the value of playing?

We've all experienced those moments of "sweet spots" in athletics. Take golf, for instance. You take your stance on the green, eyeing the direct line between your ball and the cup, and take the smallest backswing possible, gently tapping the ball. Before the ball even leaves the club's face, you know you've hit it dead center. Or take basketball, when you're standing at the free throw line focusing on the basket fifteen feet away and ten feet up. Before the ball even leaves your hands, you know it's going to be nothing but net. Or take baseball, when you're at home plate, the tip of the bat making small circles in the air just off your right ear, and you see with total clarity the spin and trajectory of the ball. You know this is going to be a hit.

Even watching these moments can be breathtaking, though I may be the only person who becomes misty-eyed during the highlight segment on Sports Center while working out on an elliptical trainer listening to Bruce

Springsteen. But I recognize that these are moments of transcendence and grace, when we know that perfection is within our grasp. The moments don't happen every time, and that is what makes each experience so memorable.

The late writer John Jerome wrote a book about this in 1980 called *The Sweet Spot in Time: The Search for Athletic Perfection.*[18] In it, Jerome explores the phenomenon of how our playing and recreation can transcend human limitations. We recognize it when it happens, yet we know so little of how and why it occurs.

What is the value of playing?

One thing we know is that play and recreation have been a part of human culture since the dawn of time. There is ample evidence that humans, as well as other species, may be hard-wired to play. It may serve some sort of adaptive purpose, helping the health and survival of the species. Or it may be something more profound, a part of our own journey to re-create ourselves in God's playful image. It may be a way we are trying to return to our roots—to return to what makes us unique among all God's creatures. It may be a way to live to our fullest potential, to explore the notion of how our bodies respond to the gift of play.

We know that play connects us to humanity in a very real and tangible way. Through play, we learn about the

---

18 Jerome, John. *The Sweet Spot in Time: The Search for Athletic Perfection*, (New York: Breakaway Books, 1999).

deepest parts of ourselves and how we respond to stress, teamwork, boundaries, integrity, and challenges. From wonderful moments of play, we take away lessons for the journey of life and, ultimately, it makes us better and more complete humans.

We also know that play connects us to ourselves. The "sweet spots"—the moments in athletics that just feel right—seem to occur when we simply get out of ourselves and let our minds and bodies become one. Play is perhaps the ultimate example of the possibilities of the mind-body connection. It draws on the human potential to achieve greatness, subsequently transcending our bodies and capabilities.

This leads to perhaps the greatest reason that play is more than merely a pastime: I believe play has a critical role in the healing journey. In my clinical experience, patients who incorporate play into their lives live longer. They also live more happily; they experience less clinical depression. And they simply live well—whether they have a chronic illness or are facing their retirement years.

It seems to make no difference whether the play is golf, bowling, tennis, throwing Frisbees or roller-skating. Whatever their choice of recreation, play has the potential to bring joy to one's life, thus the potential for valuable, physiological healing. Along the way, they discover humanity—themselves, their friends, their communities—and experience those "sweet spots" of grace and transcendence.

WISDOM OF THE BODY

Are there times when the patient knows best?

"You know I'm a dumb country boy," my patient said, grinning.

I looked at the man sitting before me. He had a fourth-grade education and was, for all intents and purposes, illiterate. Yet he had raised seven wonderful children and had adopted five others. Every one of his children had graduated from high school, and several were college graduates as well. He had twenty-four grandchildren, including his grandson he was raising himself.

"I just want to live long enough to see my 'little buddy' grow up," he said.

All of our conversations centered around that one goal: making sure that he lived to care for his grandson. But standing in his way of that goal was a major health problem: he had a serious valve abnormality of his heart as well as critical coronary artery disease.

I explained that he needed open-heart surgery that would consist of a valve replacement and a coronary bypass. I also explained that the odds of him living one year without surgery were 50 percent; the chances of living two years without surgery was less than five percent.

He listened to the overwhelming statistics and then made a firm decision. He would have a stent inserted in his coronary arteries. He declined valve surgery.

Are there times when the patient knows best?

The patient made a decision that was clearly the best he could have made for himself. Even though it went against every grain of my judgment as a clinician, I respected that kind of integrity. And I respect the outcome: more than five years later, the patient is living a full life and is raising his grandson despite all medical odds.

This is a man who always spoke of himself as a "dumb country boy," yet it is evident that he has a deep wisdom about his own body and science. He may not have "book smarts," but he has "life smarts." This man had what I call a wisdom of the body, a deep understanding of his life when placed in the context of his body and diseases that we all share.

It baffles me that some people have this innate bodily wisdom while others do not. It's not a matter of education. It is not a matter of socioeconomic class, wealth, status, or religious belief. It transcends race or ethnicity. Some people just seem to understand their bodies and how they will respond to various treatment options much better than we health care professionals do.

This innate wisdom may rub against health care professionals who come armed with science, statistics, and years of accumulated experience. When they suggest treatment options, they can become entrenched in expecting patients to follow their treatment recommendations. Some physicians will even go so far as to terminate the physician-patient relationship when a patient makes his or her own call.

Sure, there are times when patients make their own decisions that turn out poorly. All of the healthcare providers involved look at those cases with regret, hindsight, or perhaps even resentment. If they're being honest, though, they know that science can only approximate a certain reality, a certain truth. They often see through the glass darkly, and they are all reminded from time to time of how limited and fragile their knowledge can be.

The truth is that there *are* times when the patient knows best, as in this case of the grandfather. These are the times when the so-called collective wisdom of the experts is left lacking. Wise healers know that it is their job to listen to patients and to their stories. They respect their authenticity and maintain the healer-patient relationship as best they can. And wise patients, for their part, will often listen to their bodies and their life journeys and make sound decisions completely on their own.

SPARED FOR A PURPOSE

Are patients' outcomes determined by something beyond facts?

"I'm concerned," my colleague said over the phone.

He had a patient in his office that morning with some symptoms that involved his heart. The patient was minimizing his story, but my colleague was paying attention to what I call "the story behind the story." He was taking the symptoms seriously.

"Send him to me," I told my friend.

I had a vague sense that something wasn't quite right. The patient's exam and EKG were fine, and under normal circumstances, I might have ordered a stress test as the first diagnostic step. But on a hunch, I decided to admit him for a cardiac catheterization.

The results were startling: he had a critical disease of all of his coronary arteries.

The patient underwent coronary bypass surgery that very night. When he left the hospital six days later, he was ready to resume his active life.

But even more revelatory was what he said to me at his first post-operative visit. They were words that I

108

knew would determine his healing—perhaps as much, if not more than, the static facts.

"There is a message for me here in this illness and my life," he said. "Now it is my job to listen for it and live it."

Are patients' outcomes determined by something beyond facts?

In many cases, it is a patient's response to the facts that lies at the heart of recovery.

Unfortunately, some people see their survival as a random cosmic game of chance. They seem doomed to live in the past rather than in a new future. It's a serious mistake to overlook an illness as a random occurrence, just as I believe it's also a mistake to attribute every little thing to a God who sits in the heavens, pulling the strings of creation.

But some people, like this post-op patient, are astute and sensitive enough to know that something more than good technology was at play. While they often search religion for an explanation, this isn't universally the case. What *is* universally true is that they have a vague sense that their lives were spared for a purpose.

When these people survive a potentially lethal illness, it gets their attention. They realize there is something they are being asked to do, and they are determined to get the next part of their story right. Sometimes it's about new directions or relationships. Other times it's about healing the old parts of their lives that are in need of attention and nurturing. It can involve jobs and family, or it might be about how to structure their retirement. Regardless of what it's about, these are the people who find a reason—and a meaning—in their illness.

The Greeks have a word for this: *telos*. It means "direction or purpose or trajectory." Telos is about understanding that our lives are ordered by a higher purpose.

For these patients, an illness becomes a moment when people can come into their lives when they most need them. It becomes an opportunity for holiness and grace to break through. It becomes the fork in the road at which their lives are changed forever. They transcend the happenings in their lives and find themselves born again.

These are the people who do the best in the long haul. These patients who find meaning in their illness will find joy in their lives. They are transformed not only physically but also psychologically and spiritually—and it is their response that makes all the difference.

THE SABBATH OF
OUR LIVES

What does our vocation have to do with our retirement?

I hear a lot of talk about retirement from both patients and colleagues who are my age. I suppose it's a normal subject to ponder for people in their 60s. Generally, my patients who retire take one of two paths. There are some who find joy in retirement, and there are others who find misery.

Surprisingly, it seems that the quality of our years of rest is determined by the quality of our years of *work*. Those of us who successfully balance our heavy investments in work and in creative outlets outside of our jobs often find that retirement is one of the most fertile periods of life. However, for self-described "workaholics," those who exclusively define them- selves by work, diseases crop up, and they often do not have the inner reserves to overcome them. I have seen patients die within a year or two of retirement from diseases or illnesses that normally aren't terminal. They have exhausted themselves in their work at some deep level and cannot make a healthy shift from work to the Sabbath of their lives.

Unfortunately, many people wait until it's too late to make this connection between work and rest. Socrates once said about this, "The unexamined life is not worth living."[19] May this not be so for us. Let's take a look at how our work impacts our retirement.

What does our vocation have to do with our retirement?

The first consideration begins with the meaning of vocation. We often think of vocation as synonymous with occupation, but this misses a very important mark. *Occupation* is simply the job we perform to pay the bills. *Vocation* is our lives' calling.

Vocation is what provides meaning and direction. The word is derived from the Latin *vocare*, which means, "to call or be called." *Vocare* carries the deep notion that we are called by an inner or divine presence to live in a certain way. A vocation may be a job in the traditional sense, but it is often more than merely a job. It is about living the life we are called to live with total commitment and integrity.

This reminds me of an ancient Greek word, *telos*, which I mentioned in a previous chapter. *Telos* means "a

---

19   Plato, *The Apology of Socrates*, (Passerino Editore, 2017).

direction or purpose" that ultimately leads to authenticity and fulfillment. We discover our purpose when we listen to the inner voice and divine calling within each of us.

In an ideal world, our vocation and our occupation match, and we live the life for which we are destined. But if there is a mismatch and our longing is in one direction while our work takes us in another, we may be set up for a crisis in retirement years. We begin to have the sort of existential regrets about lost dreams and unfulfilled longings that can never be truly healed or replaced. That sort of regret is one of the hardest things I see patients go through, because there is no good answer except to keep searching for the real passions of their lives.

Now that we understand the meaning of vocation, let's consider how we go about discerning our vocation. I often see students make the mistake of allocating their college years to a particular type of job training. Those years should be about self-discovery and acquiring the learning tools that will serve them well, regardless of the job they choose. It is a time that should be about choosing wise mentors—people who have learned from experience how precious those early years are and how important those early decisions become—especially decisions about vocation.

Certainly, we all face the mundane or grueling realities of the workplace. But at the end of the day, it is the people who grasp the meaning of vocation who transition well from work to retirement. As their lives come to a close, they who have discovered their true vocations reap the greatest joys in their rest. In retirement, they explore their deep passions. They get a new lease on life. In many ways, they are born again.

THE
HEALTHCARE
SYSTEM

"Connection is health. And what our society does its best to disguise from us is how ordinary, how commonly attainable, health is. We lose our health—and create profitable diseases and dependences—by failing to see the direct connections between living and eating, eating and working, working and loving. In gardening, for instance, one works with the body to feed the body. The work, if it is knowledgeable, makes for excellent food. And it makes one hungry. The work thus makes eating both nourishing and joyful, not consumptive, and keeps the eater from getting fat and weak. This is health, wholeness, a source of delight."

—WENDELL BERRY, *THE BODY AND THE EARTH*

GENDER AND THE SOCIETAL CONTRACT

If society is funding the cost of educating a doctor, should society expect something in return?

Today, the admissions rate in Texas medical schools for females is approximately 53 percent, which roughly mirrors the population. At Baylor University, the admissions rate for females is even higher: 60 percent of its premedical students are female. This is a far cry from my medical school graduation in 1973, where there were only ten females in my class of two hundred physicians.

As the father of two daughters, I am glad equal opportunity has finally made it to my chosen vocation. The sharp increase in female doctors has enhanced health care tremendously. Females often bring superb intellectual skills balanced with an innate compassion and strong clinical intuition to their practices.

But more startling statistics related to gender have emerged. In 2008, I asked a team of students to present their research on gender issues in medicine, and they reported some disturbing findings: seven years after residency, 95 percent of male physicians were practicing full time. Seven years after residency, only 35 percent of women were still practicing full time.

There are diverse reasons that so few women practice full time. Some women leave due to childbearing, some to the realization of the toll that medicine can take on family and personal lives. Others leave due to downsizing or practice-sharing. The point is that many women are leaving medicine prematurely.

Even more disturbing was the finding that tuition only covers approximately 15 percent of the cost of a medical education. The rest is covered by a combination of state and federal taxes and reimbursements from patient care.

If society is funding the cost of educating a doctor, should society expect something in return?

These findings caused an uproar in my class, particularly in the context of gender differences. Some students were committed to the notion of medicine as a social contract—regardless of gender.

"It's not fair to all of us for women to enter medicine without the expectation that they'll practice full time," said one female student. "We have responsibilities beyond the physician-patient relationship."

"Right," a female concurred. "You're taking a spot that society needs. I'm committed to this for a lifetime. I want to do it all, and I will."

But other students disagreed. They ascribed to the pervasive notion today of radical individualism, in which we rarely think of what is good for those around us. Our only responsibility, as philosopher Ayn Rand would have said, is to our own needs and the god within us.

"If I'm smart enough to get into medical school, and this is still America," a female fired back, "then I'm free to do what I want."

"Yes, if I want to drop out after five years and have babies, that's my right," said another student.

I could sympathize with both of the students' perspectives.

One finding on which all of the students agreed is that none of them—neither male nor female—had any interest in working the eighty- or ninety-hour workweeks that had defined the generations of physicians before them. They were content to be contract employees of the system without the demands for nights or weekend calls. They wanted to have it all: fulfilling work, family, outside interests, and a healthy spiritual life.

Yet this expectation is problematic. If this generation of physicians limits its practices, it means other disciplines must expand to meet the demand. This kind of practice structure only adds to the shortage of doctors that is already plaguing our society. People are living longer, the baby boomers are getting older, and medical schools cannot expand at a rate fast enough to meet the needs. We are in a labor crisis in American medicine.

Regardless of our different ideas and expectations, health care remains a 24/7 responsibility. Yes, admission to medical schools should be gender, racially, and ethnically blind. For an admission committee to ask the kinds of questions that arise from these kinds of statistics could be considered a form of gender discrimination. Yet the reality of how society deals with these findings remains—and it will affect the delivery of health care for every American in the future.

THE ART OF MEDICINE

Is there an art to science?

When Albert Einstein was young, he was considered a bit on the lazy side. He would often sit around for hours, daydreaming about problems and seeking solutions outside the box of accepted theories. He called it "thought experiments."

His whimsical side remained even during the years that he worked on his greatest thought experiment, the theory of general relativity. A former landlord recalled that Einstein would sometimes burst out of his room, violin in hand, to join his pianist neighbor. Together, the duo spent afternoons immersed in the wild genius of Mozart.

From those hours lost in daydreams and music, the mathematician and physicist would go on to become one of the most creative and influential persons in the modern era. Later in his life, Einstein said that time spent in the fertile ground of the creative genius of music somehow connected him to the insights on which he was working. The combination of the sciences and arts in him literally changed our understanding of the universe.[20]

Is there an art to science?

In my experience, the best of science and clinical medicine often steps outside of the box and always has an artistic and intuitive side. Our left-brain function tends to be scientific, dry, precise, and analytical while our right-brain function tends to appreciate art, literature, music, and intuitive thinking. When these two functions are integrated, we reach our full potential as clinicians. This allows us to break the bounds of our understanding of what is normal—to take what we know of our patients and allow art to have its way.

The creative genius of science and art is evident all around us—as are the lackluster results when they are compartmentalized. Humans can, for example, write elaborate and accurate computer programs to analyze the data of human disease and come up with therapeutic treatment algorithms. Yet none of these programs can replace wisdom and creativity.

I witnessed this truth some years ago when a gifted biochemist I knew tried to transition from theory to practice. He had taught generations of medical students the intricacies of his science, which were, for many students, the bane of their existence. For some reason,

---

20 Walter Isaacson, *Einstein: His Life and Universe,* (New York: Simon and Schuster, 2007).

he decided to end his academic career and enroll in medical school. He completed a family medicine residency and went into private practice. However, despite his gifts in the sciences, he often could not correctly diagnose some of the simplest of medical conditions. His genius lay elsewhere. He simply was not wired for the *art* of medicine.

Patients also experience this relationship between science and art—or the lack thereof. Some patients try to reduce their illnesses to mounds of science, arriving with charts, printouts, boxes, and graphs. When their doctors attempt to think outside the box, these patients can get defensive and hold tightly to their masses of complex information. Their left-brain function limits their understanding that disease, wellness, health, and healing simply cannot be reduced to data. Their therapeutic options become self-limiting, and they often are left feeling frustrated with dry, sterile healthcare encounters.

In contrast, patients who have a well-developed artistic side are typically more flexible in their understanding of options that are realistic, if unconventional. They are comfortable with medicine and do not claim to be infallible.

The creative skills that characterize right-brain thinking may be instinctive to a certain degree, but we are now learning that they can also be taught and modeled. Medical schools now are offering courses in literature in which students read poetry, short stories, and essays and reflect upon them and their meaning in medicine. One medical school has developed a class on art and medicine in which students examine great works of art and integrate them into their inner lives as physicians. In the Medical Humanities program at Baylor University, this foundational shift in thinking is essential to what we are trying to teach students.

I believe we are on the cusp of some very important work. This approach of combining the sciences and arts opens the door for a whole new way of processing illness, disease, and healing. Hopefully, future generations of patients will benefit from the balanced perspective of Einstein.

A VOW OF STABILITY

How do we restore long-term relationships in health care?

Several years ago, I received an invitation to a college graduation. When I opened it, I smiled at the name printed on the card. She was my patient for twenty years and counting, and I still vividly remembered the first time I had met her.

I had been called to see her one night, just an hour after her birth. She had a heart rate of 300 beats per minute. It sounded like the wings of a hummingbird. She had such a struggle to enter the world that I could not distinguish individual heart sounds as much as a vibration. Her heart was dangerously out of rhythm; a few hours more, and her life might have been in serious jeopardy. Yet her heart responded quickly to intravenous medication, and she was stabilized.

She was the tiniest of things, not premature, but a little miniature person with an iron will to live. And live she did. After a few days, she went home and did quite well initially. Periodically, however, her electrical heart anomaly would jump out of rhythm again.

Finally, by age six, technology had advanced to the point that she underwent a surgical procedure. Her rhythm was corrected permanently, allowing her to get off her medication.

Over the years, I had continued to see her as both a patient and as a soccer player at the tournaments she played with my daughter. And now here she was, a graduate with a bright future ahead of her. I expected to see her get married and have children, thanks to the sweet stability of her health.

I can't help but notice that her story of stability is in direct contrast to the lack of stability that has become typical in the world of health care. Nearly gone are the days of long-term relationships between physicians and patients. Today, the norm is large systems and institutions employing doctors. Patients are growing up not knowing anything else but corporate medicine, where doctors are salaried employees who simply come and go and can be replaced on a whim.

We are becoming nothing more than transient problem-solvers, fixing one thing and moving on to the next. I've read that the average American has an average of 8.5 jobs in his or her working life. An average physician will have 3.5 or more practice changes. This represents a quantum shift from prior generations that is leading to major stress points in the patient-physician relationship. If we are always looking for new doctors, new patients, and new circumstances, the special long-term relationships at the bedrock of health care are at risk.

How do we restore long-term relationships in health care?

We should first recognize that it is not the government or necessarily even big business that is doing this to American medicine. It is physicians and patients who are doing it to ourselves. We seem to have forgotten that long-term healthy relationships are primarily between two human beings. We simply cannot have relationships with systems or institutions.

Restoring our long-term relationships requires intentional, hard choices by all parties, similar to the choices made by monks in ancient times. Back then, monks vowed to remain in one place for the duration of their lives. Despite the temptation to move or change because of dissatisfaction with things, they settled in for the long haul. They took vows of what was called "stability to the community." They may be ancient choices, but they are still just as relevant today.

We must value the long-term stability of forty-year relationships more than the efficiency and expediency of corporate systems. We must get involved with each other's lives and stories to strengthen the bedrock foundation of medicine. Patients and doctors alike need to speak up for meaningful relationships that stand the test of time. It is only when we forge these kinds of relationships that we can change our course.

THE VALUE OF
A HUMAN LIFE

What do we do with the outliers?

He was a young man in the prime of life. He owned a successful family business, was married to a wonderful wife, and was raising four beautiful children. But while at a family picnic, he collapsed without warning.

CPR was administered by others at the scene. By the time the ambulance arrived, he was in full-blown cardiac arrest. Drugs were administered to stabilize his cardiac rhythm, but they were unsuccessful. He was intubated and placed on life support at the scene, and CPR was continued in the ambulance on the way to the hospital. Finally, just as the ambulance arrived at the hospital he regained a semblance of a cardiac rhythm that could sustain life.

Upon arrival in the Coronary Care Unit, he was comatose. His pupils were fixed and dilated, a clinical sign of irreversible brain damage that is considered the equivalent of brain death. Just as I arrived, his rhythm again deteriorated and, again, we initiated CPR. For over an hour we struggled with a pulse that came and went. We gave him every drug in our pharmacological war chest, but we could not sustain his life. He showed no signs of responding, and we finally began to acknowledge the apparent futility of our endeavors.

The nurses, who often have infinite wisdom in these matters, looked at me with pleading eyes to stop. "Let this man die in peace," were the unspoken words I heard. When he finally flatlined, I told the nurses to stop CPR. I glanced at the clock, noting the time of death, and prepared to go to the chart and make the appropriate documentation in the medical records. There was a stillness in the room, a solemn honoring of the all-too-familiar presence of death. It is never easy for any of us in the field, but it is a part of our daily reality.

And then something happened that, to this day, is simply unexplainable.

As I left the room, I was flooded with a sense that this man's life and destiny were not yet completed. The story wasn't over. There was still work for him to do.

I walked quickly back into the room and instructed the nurses to begin CPR again and give him one more round of cardiac stimulant drugs. I injected adrenaline directly into his heart muscle instead of his IV. Just as we were about ready to once again terminate our efforts, his heart resumed pumping. It stabilized. His blood pressure started climbing, and his skin started to warm, turning from ashen blue to red. We were astonished, for none of us held one ounce of faith that we could save him.

He was placed on a ventilator overnight and, despite apparent brain death, he woke up the next day. We removed the ventilator. Two weeks later, he walked out of the hospital. This man who had been declared dead returned to work and ran his business for another twenty-five years. He saw his teenage children grow up to become successful adults on their own and lived to see his grandchildren born.

Unexplainable? Certainly. It defied everything I know and believe to be true about the human body and science. No computer simulation or therapeutic algorithm would have defined our last attempt to save his life as a "best practice pattern." His case was, in medical parlance, an "outlier"—something outside the statistical norm. What we do with these cases that are outside the norm is a question I struggle with routinely.

What do we do with the outliers?

We live in an era in which both private industry and federal policy are going to define the norms of how we treat patients. In an attempt to contain costs, we draw tight boxes around diseases and appropriate medical management. Hospitals and physicians are going to be held accountable for their decisions, and "scorecards" will be generated for the public to review and decide who is "the best doctor" based on how we all comply with well-documented science. Physicians who are "outliers" will be either fined or not reimbursed for practices that fall outside the realm of the standards. If charges exceed the predicted costs of the given diagnosis, a hospital will be penalized, or payment will be withheld. The art of medicine will give way to statistics.

While I don't necessarily have a problem with these noble attempts to rein in costs, I will say this quite honestly: I could be in a similar clinical situation again another 1,000 times, and I would never see that particular outcome in 999 of them. It defies all knowledge, all probability, and all odds. But if I felt like I did at that point in time, I would do it all the same. Even if I lost the next 999 patients. Even if meant I'd find my name on a list of doctors who do not practice by "acceptable" standards.

At the end of the day, it's not about the norms or the scorecards or the payments. It's about the value of a human life. And what *is* the value of one human life? I am not sure. But ask the family of this man, and they'll tell you what it meant to have him in their midst another twenty-five years.

LOST IN TRANSLATION

How can we make sure cultural differences don't result in bad outcomes?

A very powerful book that I've used in premedical classes for years is titled, *The Spirit Catches You and You Fall Down.*[21] It is a painfully poignant, true story of a child with epilepsy in a Hmong immigrant community in northern California. The child was under the care of a team of expert pediatricians and neurologists for many years, but there were ongoing cultural clashes between her team of healthcare experts, her family, and her extended immigrant support group.

In this child's case, the Hmong community viewed epilepsy and seizures as a divine gift, not a medical issue. In some cultures, such as theirs, epilepsy is a mark of God's favor. Therefore, they were not at all interested in making sure the child took the medicine as needed. As the seizures progressed and went untreated,

---

21 Fadimane, Anne. *The Spirit Catches You and You Fall Down: A Hmong Child, Her American Doctors, and the Collision of Two Cultures,* (New York: Farrar, Straus and Giroux, 2012).

the child began to show signs of severe and irreversible brain damage.

All sides were well-intentioned and loving people who saw the same set of facts differently. But no amount of linguistic translation seemed to make a difference in either the cultural expectations or the devastating outcome that proved to be inevitable. As is often the case when cultural gaps exist, the patient was the one who suffered.

How can we make sure cultural differences don't result in bad outcomes?

When it comes to treating patients of different languages and cultures, we can do better.

We often mistakenly think that a translator will make everything better. We assume the process and all of our decisions and outcomes will go more smoothly. Yet I have learned that providing health care for patients with different languages or cultures is not about literal translations. This was tragically illustrated in the story of the Hmong child, and it was made evident to me in medical school.

One of our cases, an elderly Hispanic female, had what is termed "failure to thrive." She was going downhill with erratic fevers, weight loss, and impending multiple organ failure. The best and brightest minds around—infectious disease specialists, oncologists, nephrologists, immunologists—were baffled. We had a Spanish speaker join us, but no amount of linguistic translation helped. The patient was dying.

Then a Hispanic ward clerk asked if she could bring in her *curandera*. Loosely translated, a *curandera* is a shaman or traditional community healer. There were some eye rolling and groans, but the wise attendant gave permission. The *curandera* spent a few hours with the patient, during which none of us were allowed to witness what transpired.

Within twenty-four hours, the patient began to feel better. Lab values normalized. Fevers abated. Kidney failure was averted. A few days later, she walked out of the hospital.

All of us were humbled, awed, and intellectually perplexed. We wanted rational, scientific explanations, and of course we had none. We were merely silent witnesses to the phenomenal healing of a woman who was raised from the dead in every sense of the word except the literal. The *curandera* touched upon something deep, timeless, and beyond quantification. It was the ability of one person to be an agent of grace, exposing the patient and healer to depths that we had difficulty understanding.

It became clear to me that cultural differences run deeper than language. In order to properly meet the needs of non-English speakers, physicians need more than translators. They need to learn about the culture in which their patients serve and live. They need to learn how cultural forces shape and define patients' lives. The worst outcomes can be avoided when physicians put aside their own cultural assumptions, backgrounds, and experiences. Healing can happen when they give a bit of effort to understanding the lives of their patients.

We saw a physician do this successfully in the classic television series, *Northern Exposure.*[22] The main character was a Jewish physician from the Northeast named Dr. Joel Fleischman, who found himself practicing medicine in a small, remote Alaskan village. It was filled with an odd and humorous collection of residents. Dr. Fleischman was often out of his cultural element, yet his openness to learning new ways enabled him to relate to an environment foreign to the one in which he was trained.

We can meet the needs of patients from different cultures if we are willing to adopt the same openness as this fictional doctor. We are a melting pot in the United States, historically and today, which is both a strength of our country and a challenge for physicians. A rural southerner, for example, may have different worldviews, language quirks, and expectations of the healthcare system than a sophisticated urban resident. A Hispanic man may have a different set of needs than an urban black man, while an urban black man may have a different set of expectations than a female Muslim immigrant. We need to be understanding and sensitive to every patient's background.

Our job is to give the best health care that we know how to provide to the human being before us. Period.

---

22 *Northern Exposure.* Created by Joshua Brand and John Falsey. CBS, 1990-1995.

No other option is acceptable. To deliver adequate health care, we need to remove ourselves from a public policy debate that has become a political quagmire. And while the economics of that are for the voters and politicians to ultimately decide, it is also up to us to stand up for any and all patients who come to us for our services.

Our historic mandate is to be agents of healing. That has not changed in a millennium, and it is my hope that it never will.

THE MISSING
GENERATION

How do we handle older generations who are raising youth?

My patient was in her early 70s and feeling tired and run down. Her husband had been a patient of mine through two bypass surgeries, and now she was in my clinic with a pulse rate between 30 to 40 beats per minute. It was clear that she needed a pacemaker.

But she didn't wait to hear about risks or benefits. She didn't ask about cost. She didn't ask all the normal questions that are asked before getting a pacemaker. There was only one thing she wanted to know.

"Will it give me enough stamina to raise my five-year-old granddaughter?" she asked.

I studied her for a moment. "Well, there's no pacemaker I know of that'll give you what you need to raise a teenage girl," I said, then added with a smile, "but that I think the pacer will at least get you *ready* for those years."

This scenario is happening with increasing frequency in medical offices nationwide. Patients in their fifth, sixth, and even seventh decades are raising another generation of children in the absence of the children's parents, to whom I refer as the "missing generation." The causes of the absenteeism of this missing generation are complex and diverse. Some parents are away due to military assignments, divorce, or job transfers. Others are gone due to substance abuse, incarceration, or economic devastation.

But the cause isn't the point. The point is that parents are missing. And the common denominator is that the elder generation is now raising a whole new family. A generation of patients that should be entering retirement years now has to bear the responsibility for the health, education, and well-being of these youth. The stresses this causes are enormous.

What strikes me is not that this happens. Life can throw us all curve balls. What affects me is the grace with which these patients bear this burden. They carry the stresses with strength and quiet dignity. I have never heard a word of complaint from any of my patients about their reality, even when their health, financial stability, or retirement plans are touched. They are true heroes of a society that is undergoing shifts in demographics and family structures.

And, of course, these dynamics have very real ramifications for the healthcare team. Health issues for the older couple are often magnified by the stresses that are placed on their lives. Not only that, but decisions about their health issues, treatment options, drug costs, and prognoses have to be filtered through their reality.

It's further complicated by the fact that insurance and Medicare issues become increasingly complex. And if the children have health issues of their own and legal guardianship has not been addressed, they often fall between the cracks of financial coverage.

How do we handle older generations who are raising youth?

The discussion as to how to manage the healthcare needs of all of the parties in this situation has financial, political, and moral parameters.

On one extreme, some people argue that the government has no stake in this problem—that it's up to families to fend for themselves. If insurance is denied to any of the extended family, they say it's the problem of the family. They believe it is a commercial transactional problem and that health care is simply one more commodity on the marketplace to be bought and sold, with no real-world moral ramifications for society at large. In this model, there is no room for compassion or virtue. Each of us sinks or swims as we are able. It is social Darwinism, and only the strongest, wealthiest, and most able will survive. This thinking is the ultimate outcome of the Ayn Rand pseudo-philosophy embraced by many politicians in these complex times.

On the other side of the ideological spectrum, some people see this as a microcosm of a larger issue in society and that any solution must take society into account.

They believe that these problems affect the productivity and stability of society and that we must all pull together to protect those who are most vulnerable.

While these extremes may be rare, both are surely a reality for some in the public and political arenas as well as the personal and private sectors. This is our reality as physicians and as a society. We live in an imperfect world amid forces of darkness that have the potential to undermine our way of practicing the healing arts that has been foundational for thousands of years.

Ultimately, the care of our patients must factor in the holistic realities of their lives. Decisions are never made in a vacuum, and resources are never allocated in ways that will be fair to all. We must find a system that works for all, that is as fair as possible to all, and is financially prudent as a society. It is an investment in our productivity as a nation, and to do less is a moral failure of the highest order.

And while we may sign contracts with the government, with various insurance carriers, and with the hospitals that may well be our employers and "bosses," at the end of the day, I believe our best way to handle this situation is to remember to whom we have a moral responsibility. Our covenant is with our patients. They, and they alone, must be our guiding star.

SHIFT PHYSICIANS

Does limiting work shifts make better doctors?

When Congress adopted legislation limiting the workweek for medical interns and residents to eighty hours, my first thought was, "Where was this law when I needed it?"

During my years of internship and residency, going home wasn't an option when I was on call. Back then, I learned how to function in spite of ongoing sleep deprivation. I enjoyed quiet times in evenings with patients and families, and I discovered that a few hours of full-court basketball after working thirty-six hours can be therapeutic, especially when followed by pizza and beer.

The new legislation aimed to reduce the fatigue factor in training programs. Studies had indicated that some medical mistakes were directly attributable to long hours, exhaustion, and poor communication among staff, and so the limited workweek was passed with the best of intentions. The hope was that mistakes would be minimized and patient care would be improved.

Then further limitations to the eighty-hour work week were proposed. The Accreditation Council for

Graduate Medical Education published a recommendation in *The New England Journal of Medicine*[23] that would mandate that first-year residents work no longer than a sixteen-hour shift and have constant supervision. More senior residents would work no longer than a twenty-four-hour shift.

Does limiting work shifts make better doctors?

It all sounds reasonable and good on paper, and certainly patient safety should be of paramount importance. There is only one problem with this noble objective: there's no evidence that it works.

Data gathered after the first regulation went into effect hasn't supported claims that shorter workweeks translate to improved patient care. There has been no meaningful reduction in medical errors since the eighty-hour week was mandated. Some even claim that mistakes may be slightly higher.

One reason that errors remain a problem is that the more we become shift physicians, the greater the likelihood for communication mistakes to develop between staff who inherit the patients from their colleagues who are rotating off duty. In other words, the more "hand offs" of relaying clinical information and data from one member of the team to another, the more often mistakes occur.

---

23 *The New England Journal of Medicine*, (Massachusetts: Massachusetts Medical Society, 1812-present).

Why? Because people seem to have this infuriating habit of getting deathly sick at any hour. Human bodies don't recognize holidays, work schedules, or outside commitments. Illness is unpredictable. Transmission of data either verbally or via computer cannot tell a story of an iron will to live nor a family that is being rent asunder. The more we divide patient care and continuity among smaller and smaller parcels of physicians and specialists, none of whom communicate with each other as well they should, the more errors can happen. Physician fatigue is certainly real, but imposing federal guidelines to reduce this has simply not addressed the unintended consequences that can occur.

A second consequence of this part of healthcare training is a growing rate of dissatisfaction and early burnout among young physicians. All medical schools are aware of this trend and are searching for ways to prevent this in young graduates. While all might not agree with this conclusion, I feel that physicians who have not entered the crucible of loss and pain with their patients are particularly prone to a malaise of the soul. Without embracing the pain that comes from this, they also fail to seek and find the glorious joy that medicine can become. They become contract shift workers, instead of partners embracing a holy calling and vocation. I find it more than curious that as the weekly demands of post-graduate medical education were implemented, the satisfaction rate of physicians sank to an all-time low. Burnout, emotional fatigue, clinically reported rates of depression, and suicides by young physicians have risen to an all-time high. One would think that by lowering the physical demands of medical education, the converse would be true. We should be seeing a happier, healthier, and more fulfilled group of physicians. And we are not.

A third and final unintended consequence of this new regulation is that we have now succeeded in training a generation of physicians who have little experience in crisis medicine. By functioning primarily as shift physicians, they have less experience when a patient crisis erupts. Our system of care seems to be moving to delivery models of outpatient wellness care and inpatient sick care. But the skillsets that are necessary to manage the two models are fundamentally different and, ultimately, complementary. I firmly believe that even if one wants to practice only outpatient "shift" medicine, he or she should also have a deep working knowledge of the impact of inpatient care and tragedy not only on patients' lives but on the physician's own life as well.

The system is fundamentally flawed because limiting work shifts doesn't seem to get to the heart of the matter. When patients become sick enough to require hospitalization, they need someone to attend to them who knows their case. And when crises come, young physicians need to have honed their skillsets so that they can respond appropriately. Until we address these deeper systemic issues, it seems that focusing on the work schedules of physicians-in-training is a bit like plugging a dike with a pinkie finger and expecting the water to stop leaking.

DUST TO DUST

Should we preserve life at all costs?

"You are dying," my pastor said firmly. He looked around the room at those of us gathered on Ash Wednesday. "You are dying. And the only difference is that some of you know it and have been given a specific diagnosis and a general timeline, and others of you don't. But rest assured: it is happening." As we stepped forward to have ashes rubbed on our foreheads, he added solemnly, "Remember that you are dust, and to dust you shall return." We filed out of the church in silence and darkness.

His forceful words intended to shock us out of our complacency, and they did. Even more startling, I was reminded again of our shared fate just two days later.

I received a tender, quiet email from a colleague at Baylor University who was diagnosed recently with terminal pancreatic cancer. He said he may have six months left to live, and he wanted to thank me for a workshop I led at his church many years ago. I had walked the pastoral care team through the major difference between healing and curing. Healing, I had reminded them, is possible even as we walk through the valley of the shadow of death. It is possible when curing is painfully absent.

In words that were so typical of the sweet, gentle man I knew him to be, I saw courage in the face of darkness and love in the place of despair. I saw his acceptance of the words that I heard my pastor say only two nights before. *Yes, I am dying*, he said to me.

He did not rage at the injustice of it all. He didn't place his life on an idolatrous altar. He didn't choose technology over compassion, dignity, or God. He didn't extend his life at all costs. My friend chose only the very basic palliative care and would go quite gently into the good night. I was sure that he would die with the peace and dignity with which he lived.

Should we preserve life at all costs?

In my experience, our individual responses to our inevitable passing seem to depend on our education levels and socioeconomic standards. In forty years of medicine, I have observed that the most aggressive and unending treatment options are often chosen by those who have been pushed to the margins most of their lives. The people who have been the most disenfranchised by medicine often want "everything done," even when the medical team knows it is wasted effort.

Often, the higher the education and socioeconomic level of the patient, the more he or she wants to simply die with minimal heroic measures. This observation was confirmed when, later that same week, I received yet *another* reminder about our fate.

A dozen or more friends forwarded an article published in the *Wall Street Journal* that was titled, "Why Doctors Die Differently." The gist of the article was the rather amazing and very true statement that doctors—who surely have access to the latest clinical and research trials and cutting-edge technology—often forgo these treatments when faced with terminal illness. They tend to choose to die simply and quietly, surrounded by loved ones. No heroic measures. No extended treatment plans that more often than not result in only more suffering. No life support in terminal and futile situations. They just let be what will be.[24]

Within one week, I had heard essentially the same story from three different sources and through three different lenses. And they all came to the same conclusion: we are dying. My pastor, my friend, and other doctors freely acknowledge that we are dust, and to dust we shall return.

Allowing ourselves to die with dignity is something that most people could agree is a good thing. It is something that most religious traditions hold in common. But living up to that reality becomes hard for us in times of crisis when emotions are running high.

As we weigh the costs of preserving life or submitting to death, let us begin with a simple, humble

---

24 Ken Murray. "Why Doctors Die Differently," *The Wall Street Journal*, February 25, 2012.

admission of our own finitude. We must face the fact that we live our biological lives in a sort of Lent, and we face a shared mortality. It is Lent, and to dust we shall return.

TIPTOEING AROUND FISCAL ACCOUNTABILITY

What can be done about national healthcare spending?

When it comes to end-of-life decisions and expenditures, the circumstances and conversations are never easy. They raise fundamental political and spiritual questions for our families—*and* for our society.

Take, for example, a 90-year-old man with advanced Alzheimer's disease who lives in an assisted living center. He no longer recognizes his family. He is bed-bound. He has to be fed, bathed, and cleaned daily. He had two pacemakers inserted when he was younger, and now his last one is wearing out. The family must decide whether they will request a battery replacement so that their father can continue to live another six or seven years. If they do, society will foot the bill through Medicare. If they do not, some will consider it an immoral decision; others will consider it illegal.

Or consider an 85-year-old patient who develops kidney failure. Already an amputee, she is bedridden. She is reasonably alert, and her family enjoys her presence. Without dialysis, she will die within weeks. But committing to dialysis carries enormous risks, not to mention the grim reality of ongoing weekly treatments that take a toll. Because dialysis is a federally-funded and mandated procedure, there will be no choice but to proceed if her family demands it.

Cases like these play out daily in medical offices and hospitals across the country, yet no one is asking about the ultimate cost of these treatments. Patients, families, and providers are prolonging human life at the expense of simple dignity—the triumph of technology over judgment, as a wise physician calls it. Meanwhile, healthcare reform discussions tiptoe around this most important issue to the future of our country.

As a nation, we are refusing to accept the many realities we face when we are dying. An alarming set of data confirms that twenty-five percent of our national healthcare expenditures are incurred in the last thirty days of life *when we know the outcome is futile*. We continue to insist that all diseases can be conquered and that death can be squelched. We think we can avoid our certain fate if only we pour enough resources into health care. Our minds tell us otherwise, of course, and deep down, we must certainly know better.

The disastrous consequence is that we are squandering precious resources. We already have the resources to provide a reasonable, fundamental quality of health care for all our citizens. It would not require new programs or higher taxes as some might expect, but it would require some collective action on our part.

What can be done about national healthcare spending?

I believe proper allocation of our resources begins with honesty. We must be honest with ourselves about our finitude. A life that is well lived and a death that occurs with dignity and grace are perhaps all any of us could ask for.

With this humble perspective, perhaps we can come to the collective conclusion that life is not the ultimate virtue. Together, we can shift our healthcare goals. The ultimate goal of health care, then, becomes not about the preservation of life at all costs but about compassion, competence, and love. This allows patients, families, and providers to admit when technology has run its course. It allows them to calmly and collectively say that prolonging human life at the expense of simple dignity is no longer advisable.

It also means that there are limitations to what society is willing to do and fund—and that our spending should be accountable to those limitations. As taxpayers, we have the right to demand that our dollars are well spent. The director of Health and Human Services under President George W. Bush, Michael Leavitt, believed that the government has every right to ask questions about the appropriate treatment for which the government was paying. In the same way that we don't want to pay $2,000 for a hammer for the military, we should demand the same sort of fiscal accountability of our health care system. Leavitt believed that government should be fiscally prudent and conservative in its spending of federal dollars.

Ultimately, we must be willing to have a calm, respectful, national conversation about rationing health care. When other administrations have raised the same concerns as Leavitt, there has been outrage and unfounded allegations about government takeover of medicine. We should be able to talk without one side accusing the other of "death panels," inflammatory rhetoric, and threats of catastrophe or socialism. Yes, we must be cautious about turning these decisions over to congressional committees and legislation. Yes, we must not leave these decisions to corporate boardrooms and stockholders. And yes, we must be careful about turning a blind eye and saying, "Let's leave it to the marketplace and the sanctity of the physician-patient relationship." But we cannot continue to avoid the reality that we have abundant healthcare resources that we are not using wisely.

Let us face these issues together and wisely, or surely we will all fail together in our efforts to provide compassionate care for our society.

THE VIRTUES OF MEDICINE

What is the Christian model for health care?

Several years ago, I was invited to speak at Belmont University by Dr. Todd Lake, the former chaplain at Baylor University. The title of the lecture he asked me to give was "Christian Health Care." At first glance, I thought it would be relatively easy to put it together. After all, I come from a Christian background and perspective, and I practice in a community that has two faith-based hospitals. I felt pretty well-qualified to speak on this particular topic.

But the deeper I studied the topic, the harder and more elusive it became. I found myself with more questions than answers. For example, how does one even begin to define the terms "Christian health care"? Does a Christian healthcare system necessarily embody the teachings of Jesus? Also, can a healthcare provider who claims to be a follower of Christ—yet who refuses to provide care for the indigent or Medicare and Medicaid patients—be labeled a "Christian physician"? Can a devout gentle Muslim or

Hindu who gives his or her time to health care for the poor, like many of my premedical students do, be considered an anonymous "Christian" (a term used in some theological literature)? And can a country that rushes to proclaim its Christian heritage in an election year—and then ignores the reality of 25 percent of its population—truly and honestly lay claim to its Christian beliefs?

These questions drove me deep into the wells of my beliefs and practice. The answers that emerged are what I shared in my lecture at Belmont University. I presented them with full understanding of the fact that they may not have been popular ideas back then, and I'm presenting them again here with the understanding that they may not be popular now. Nonetheless, I invite you to reflect on these simple observations about "Christian health care" that have been gleaned from forty years of practicing medicine in both faith-based and private, for-profit hospitals.

Let's start with an understanding of the term "Christian." As it pertains to the delivery of good health care, Christian faith must embody more than a set of doctrinal beliefs or mission statements. It has to be more than a charter and a tax status. It must be a living, breathing model upon which to encounter human brokenness.

Now let's consider the individuals and institutions around us through this lens of Christian faith. Some faith-based hospitals and systems apply this model well; others do not. That is reality. Some for-profit hospitals and systems do this well; others do not. That is reality. Some physicians embody the teachings of Jesus but would be appalled at being labeled Christians. Others claim to be followers of Christ and are dysfunctional human beings driven by profit and greed. That is also reality. Some totally secular western industrialized countries embody what I would consider Christian practices and yet are decidedly not Christian. And some countries that proclaim such faith are models of corruption and corporate greed. Talk about ambiguity!

What is the Christian model for health care?

I told my audience at Belmont University that to be considered a "Christian" model for health care, a healthcare provider or institution should give more than lip service to three cardinal virtues.

1. Compassion

Simply put, a system or provider must care deeply about what he is doing and how he or she does it. Compassion literally means "to suffer with." In other words, we must be willing to take the suffering of our patients and their loved ones seriously. We must listen to their stories and walk with them through the confusing myriad of options they face. Compassion is more than an emotional feeling. It is a movement that forces us to act in certain ways that are consistent with our proclaimed beliefs. It is not a touchy-feely, naïve sense of concern, but a moral compass that moves us to actions based on a lived community of faith and a vibrant intellectual heritage.

2. Wisdom

This is different than wielding facts with power and success. And it doesn't mean having all the answers. Wisdom is about being good stewards of our resources. We are called to be financially conservative and accountable for our future while we provide the health care that we know we have the power and knowledge to deliver. Fortunately, it has nothing at all to do with a given religious belief system. Some physicians have innate wisdom at a young age; others never will. It can be modeled and taught, but until it is lived, it is nothing but chaff in the wind. And just as individuals are called to wisdom, systems and governments are also called to an accountability based on the virtue of wisdom.

3. Justice.

From a Biblical sense and through the eyes of Jesus, justice is more than a sense of fair play. It is more than a casual glance at the vision statement of a system. Justice embodies the very notion of the Judeo-Christian understanding of God and God's kingdom. One writer said it succinctly: "Biblical justice involves making individuals, communities, and the cosmos whole by upholding goodness and impartiality." Healing—which is in what we are called to participate—is always grounded in justice. True healing in this sense is not about curing nor is it about the indiscriminate use of science. It is about wholeness of the human condition, and it applies to all. If we as healers are to embody these virtues as the tides of medicine change, I think it will take more than using common terms such as "Christian health care." It will require a whole different understanding and use of language and ideas. May we each dig deep into the wells of our shared faith traditions as Americans to develop a living, breathing model of health care in a broken world. Moving forward, may our model embody the hope, compassion, and a respect for the whole individual that is called for in these rapidly changing times.

A LETTER TO THE
NEXT GENERATION

Dear Reader,

On Christmas day in 2013, I completed my last forty-eight-hour shift as a cardiologist. It had been forty years of nights and weekend calls, and on that day, I let go of that responsibility and transitioned into retirement.

I felt it fitting and highly symbolic to work that holiday, inserting pacemakers and stents into those who were truly in need. Many of those in need were, for me, a modern-day version of an unwed, pregnant homeless mother two thousand years ago searching for a place to birth her child. A few had health coverage in one capacity or another; many did not. All received the same standard of care by our hospitals and the best of technology. For that, I was proud of our community.

As I pondered the years of retirement that lie ahead of me, I found myself standing at a crossroads of exhilaration and grieving. I had taught my students that doctors are prone to identity confusion; more often than in many professions, we confuse our work with our essence. Surely, I had told them, who we are is something fundamentally different than what we do every day. Yet I realized that being a physician is so deeply rooted in my being. I knew I was heading into deep waters.

It has been deep waters indeed. As I travel new roads to self-discovery, I am being led to new joys found in new freedoms. There is still so much wonder in the world that I want to taste and discover. I am excited about experiencing the final stages of a life that has been blessed in so many ways.

At the same time, I am also experiencing a form of grief, for I miss medicine every day. I am losing a part of myself that I know I may never get back. In many ways, it is—as I have written—a form of death. The old self is dying, and I am not totally sure what kind of self will take its place, which is, of course, the same spiritual paradox in which we all find ourselves when we live long enough. We must die to ourselves in order to be born again.

From my own personal crossroads, I find that it is not unlike the crossroads at which our healthcare system now stands.

You see, during the incredible span of time that I was in medicine, there was much reason to be exhilarated. I saw the dawn of technology with which patients were afforded procedures and devices that were not in anyone's imagination when I began. I saw the birth of computers and imaging change our fundamental understanding of disease and how we diagnose and treat the neediest of our patients. I saw electronic medical records supplant simple listening and the human touch. I saw the infancy of gene manipulation and its endless possibilities for our common good.

Yet there has also been much to grieve about health care. As the science and technology have exploded, there has been an inverse curve in our understanding of the nature of the human condition. Students and residents have become extremely good at ordering tests and prescribing new medications but do not yet have the gift of wisdom in knowing when to implement them. We've been generating sterile and meaningless reports in order to code at higher reimbursement levels. Over time, we have become impoverished caretakers of the human soul and spirit, confusing good science with mature reasoning and compassion. Our health care has failed us on so many levels.

And so we find ourselves fragmented, lost, wandering in the desert of our moral and scientific landscape. We are thirsty, and the streams from which we are drinking are not sustaining us. If we don't find our way back home, we will certainly lose the precious gift we were bequeathed by those gone before us.

Providers and consumers alike are hopelessly frustrated, bewildered, and at times angry. Some of us complain that the insurance companies are ruining the good side of medicine; some blame the government. While there is certainly some truth to these claims, it only touches on a deeper and more fragile side of medicine. And in many areas, we have no one to blame but ourselves. When we had a chance to stand up for our patients against the onslaught of outside forces, we were silent. We sought ever-increasing ways to maximize profits; we became slave traders of technology.

Today, we are in a time of crisis and transition. The world of medicine in which I grew up no longer exists, but there must be a better way than our current way of administering health care.

And so, for all of the glory and wonder of medicine, it is now time to pass the torch to you, the next generation of healers and patients. It is your job and legacy to fill the shoes and lives of the ones that have gone before you. In many ways, you are a blank slate. You are not colored by the memories of the "good old days," so you have the opportunity to creatively adapt to change. I believe you can impact the direction of health care in our country in four ways: learning, mentoring, listening, and, most of all, loving.

Learning

For starters, you should learn something of the various economic models of healthcare delivery so that you don't succumb to the simplistic, reductionist sound bites of politicians and the media. But I believe we make a mistake when we only focus on economic problems and solutions . . . It goes deeper than that. We somehow have to grow into our understanding of medicine as an art—a holy and timeless calling that sustains both the healer and the patient.

We need to go back in time and history to a more fundamental understanding of human nature. To do this, I believe all premedical students should be immersed in the world of humanities as well as science. You should be exposed to the myriad of lovely short stories that abound of illness. You should read poetry by both patients and physicians. You should learn some of the classical philosophical underpinnings of medicine and their impact on its history. You should learn to look at art with an inner eye so that you can see the same images in the wounded patients you encounter. Mainly, we should learn something about ourselves in a very real, deep, and mysterious way.

In a practical way, medical schools are in the infancy of passing on this kind of understanding of how the roots of medicine have shaped us. We should always cherish and demand a dedication to scientific truth and disciplined integrity, and we should draw from the deep well of narrative experiences that have preceded the scientific revolution by millennium. At Baylor University, we honed in on this many years ago with the belief that a student is "formed" by his or her undergraduate years. Long before the demands of medical school and residency come speeding into your soul like a runaway locomotive and you switch into a survival mode, choose to shape your way of interpreting the world through both the sciences *and* the humanities.

Mentoring

Seek wise mentors. Most of what I have learned in medicine, I have learned from gentle and wise mentors combined with gracious and forgiving patients. The art of mentoring has shaped our culture and given us a moral compass on which to navigate strange waters. It has undergirded various models of health care from purely socialistic to highly profit-driven and purely capitalistic models. Yes, I have certainly learned from textbooks, journals, scientific sessions, and collegial work performed in the heat of battle, yet historically, mentoring at the bedside has sustained me, and it has sustained this profession.

Listening

Some of the boundaries that were taught to my generation need to be discarded. "Don't become emotionally involved with your patients," they said. "Don't show your feelings. Don't cry. Be objective." The physicians who have bought into that model are often the very ones who are most distraught about the impending changes in health care.

The truth is that our patients have something to teach us that is far more valuable than the technology we bring to the table. In teaching us about themselves, they teach us about ourselves. What more can we ask of any work?

So, quiet your heart and open your mind. Listen to stories of health care. Sit at the bedside. Talk to the staff when a crisis or mundane problem interrupts a crazy schedule. Because, at its heart, medicine is about storytelling. There are things that cannot be taught any other way.

Listening requires courage, for it requires you to be vulnerable with your patients. It takes you out of the classroom, out from hiding behind the computer screen, and into the vast spaces of wounds, pain, suffering, and redemption and grace. This is where you face your own limitations and frailties in order to help your patients with their own. This is where you become opened up to your own wounds.

Some of you will get a taste of this "realness" of medicine and know you can't live without it.

Others of you, on the other hand, will not want to experience it. I understand your fear. But those of you who live only with the fear miss the boat containing the joy. It is my firm belief that we need to confront our shadow sides to find our wholeness.

Loving

This is the most important of all. Healers have to love their patients despite a system that seems incapable of love. They have to (gasp) love their colleagues even when they disagree. They have to love themselves enough to suffer, for like it or not, we are engaged in a vocation of suffering and loss. This is our chosen lot, and it is ours to define by how well we respond to the innumerable challenges.

Thank you for listening to these stories that I've shared with you here in *Medicine at the Crossroads*. They are only a speck of dust in the infinitude of stories that are ready for us at the bedside, but they give a glimpse into the rhythm and glory of health care. They are fragments of a stained glass window, brought together as a reminder that we are a living part of tradition that embodies the very best of what it means to be a human created in the image of God.

And medicine *is* the very best. For all of the issues with our healthcare system, not once did I ever regret my choice of profession. There were days that I came home from work exhausted, drained, angry, and wounded. There were days I felt scarred and bloody and fearful for my patients. There were days I felt depleted to the point where I wasn't sure I could survive. Yet medicine remains the most amazing thing I can imagine a human being doing with his or her life. I am forever thankful for the opportunity to be a part of an ongoing miracle in so many lives.

At the end of the day, I remain hopeful, for I sense that despite all of the impending changes, I know that you, patients and healers of good, will carry the day. You can and should insist on a better world of medicine.

It is your time.

Michael Attas

BIBLIOGRAPHY

Alcoholics Anonymous World Services, *Twelve Steps and Twelve Traditions*, (New York: AA Worldwide Services, 2002), 83-87: https://www.aa.org/assets/en_US/en_step9.pdf.

Boff, Leonardo. *Sacraments of Life: Life of Sacraments*, (Oregon: Pastoral Press, 1998).

Buber, Martin. *I and Thou*, (New York: Scribner, 1978).

Cousins, Norman. *Anatomy of an Illness as Perceived by the Patient: Reflections on Healing and Regeneration*, (New York: Bantam Books, 1981).

Donne, John. "Meditation XVII: No Man is an Island," *Devotions upon Emergent Occasions*, (England, 1624).

Fadimane, Anne. *The Spirit Catches You and You Fall Down: A Hmong Child, Her American Doctors, and the Collision of Two Cultures*, (New York: Farrar, Straus and Giroux, 2012).

Fischer, Kathleen. *Winter Grace: Spirituality and Aging*, (Tennessee: Upper Room, 1998).

Flexner, Alexander. *Medical Education in the United States and Canada: A Report to The Carnegie Foundation for the Advancement of Teaching*, (New York: Carnegie Foundation, 1910).

Isaacson, Walter. *Einstein: His Life and Universe*, (New York: Simon and Schuster, 2007).

Jerome, John. *The Sweet Spot in Time: The Search for Athletic Perfection*, (New York: Breakaway Books, 1999).

Kubler-Ross, Elizabeth. *On Death and Dying*, (New York: Scribner, 1997).

Mohrmann, Margaret. *Pain Seeking Understanding: Suffering, Medicine, and Faith*, (Ohio: Pilgrim Press, 1999).

Murray, Ken. "Why Doctors Die Differently," *The Wall Street Journal*, February 25, 2012.

Name withheld by request, "It's Over, Debbie," *Journal of the American Medical Association*, 1988, as accessed April 25, 2018, at www.mclean.k12.ky.us/docs/Its%20Over%20Debbie.pdf.

New American Standard Bible, 1995.

Northern Exposure. Created by Joshua Brand and John Falsey. CBS, 1990-1995.

Plato, *The Apology of Socrates*, (Passerino Editore, 2017).

The New England Journal of Medicine, (Massachusetts: Massachusetts Medical Society, 1812-present).

Thomas, Dylan. "Do Not Go Gentle Into the Good Night," *In Country Sleep*, (New York: New Directions, 1952).

Shem, Samuel. *House of God*, (Pennsylvania: Richard Marek Publishers, 1978).

Wolterstorff, Nicholas. *Lament for a Son*, (Michigan: William B. Eerdmans Publishing Company, 1987).

Worthington, Everett, et al. "Forgiveness in Health Research and Medical Practice," *Explore: The Journal of Science and Healing*, no. 3 (May 2005): 169-176, https://doi.org/10.1016/j.explore.2005.02.012.

ABOUT THE AUTHOR

Michael Attas, MDiv, MD, didn't choose medicine so much as it chose *him*.

He was a football player and Psychology student at Baylor University when he applied for a summer job at Baylor College of Medicine. At the time, the college was looking for a student to research the cause of mysterious "mumps" appearing on patients following open heart surgery, and Attas was looking for a way out of a construction job that was planned for that summer. He had no background or interest in medicine, but because no one else applied, he got the job.

Not only did Attas discover the cause of the temporary condition; his findings were published in a national medical journal that fall. His medical intuition caught the attention of renowned heart surgeon Dr. Denton Cooley, who put his hand on Attas' shoulder on the last day of the job and said, "Mike, you have a gift. Go to medical school."

So he did. It was the start of a prominent and fulfilling career in medicine for Dr. Attas.

With a bachelor of science in psychology under his belt, he went on to earn his medical degree from The University of Texas Medical Branch in Galveston. He completed his residency and fellowship training at the University of Kentucky Medical Center where he also served as Chief Resident in the Department of Medicine and Senior Cardiology Fellow.

Board certified by the American Board of Internal Medicine with a subspecialty in cardiovascular disease, Dr. Attas practiced for forty years. He is a fellow of the American College of Cardiology and served on the Board of Directors of the McLennan County Medical Education & Research Foundation. He is also a member of the American Heart Association, the Texas Medical Society, and the McLennan County Medical Society.

Alongside his career in medicine, Dr. Attas earned a Master of Divinity with an emphasis in ethics and moral theology from the Episcopal Theological Seminary of the Southwest. He was an ordained priest and served as an assisting priest at St. Paul's Episcopal Church in Waco, Texas. He also served on the Board of Trustees of the Seminary of the Southwest and the Episcopal Health Foundation.

In 1999, Dr. Attas combined his passions for medicine and divinity to found and direct the Medical Humanities program at Baylor University, which offers a bachelor of arts for undergraduate pre-medical students. It is designed to foster an understanding of the spiritual, ethical, economic, and literary aspects of health care. The program was the first of its kind in the nation, and it continues to pave the way for other universities.

He has also taught at the University of Texas Southwestern Medical Center in Dallas, the Department of Medicine at Texas A&M University Health Science Center, Baylor College of Medicine, the University of Wyoming College of Human Medicine & Family Practice Residency Center, and the University of Colorado Medical School.

Dr. Attas has been recognized with the Ashbel Smith Distinguished Alumnus Award (UTMB, 2015) and the Lifetime Meritorious Achievement Award in Health Care (Baylor University, 2015).

Medicine at the Crossroads is his second book. It is a collection of articles that was written as a bi-weekly column on contemporary healthcare issues for the *Waco Tribune-Herald* (2009-2011). His first book, *Fly-Fishing—The Sacred Art* (SkyLight Paths Publishing, 2012), was co-authored with Rabbi Eric Eisenkramer to share lessons from fly-fishing on reflection, solitude, community, and the search for the Divine. He is also the author of several articles published in various medical journals and reviews.

Today, Dr. Attas is immensely enjoying retirement with his wife, Gail. He is no longer active in ministry, devoting his time instead to traveling and fly-fishing. He has three adult children: Jason, Jessica, and Amanda.

Dr. Attas is available for consulting and public speaking engagements for hospitals, health systems, and corporate boards involved with the healthcare industry and sector. You can reach him at michael_attas@msn.com.

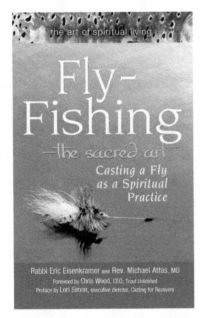